DIVERTICULITIS COOKBOOK

Discover 1800 Days of Quick and Soothing Recipes to Revitalize Your Gut and Enjoy a 45-Day Meal Plan for Lasting Relief.

Maggie Woods

TABLE OF CONTENTS

CHAPTER 1: UNDERSTANDING DIVERTICULITIS

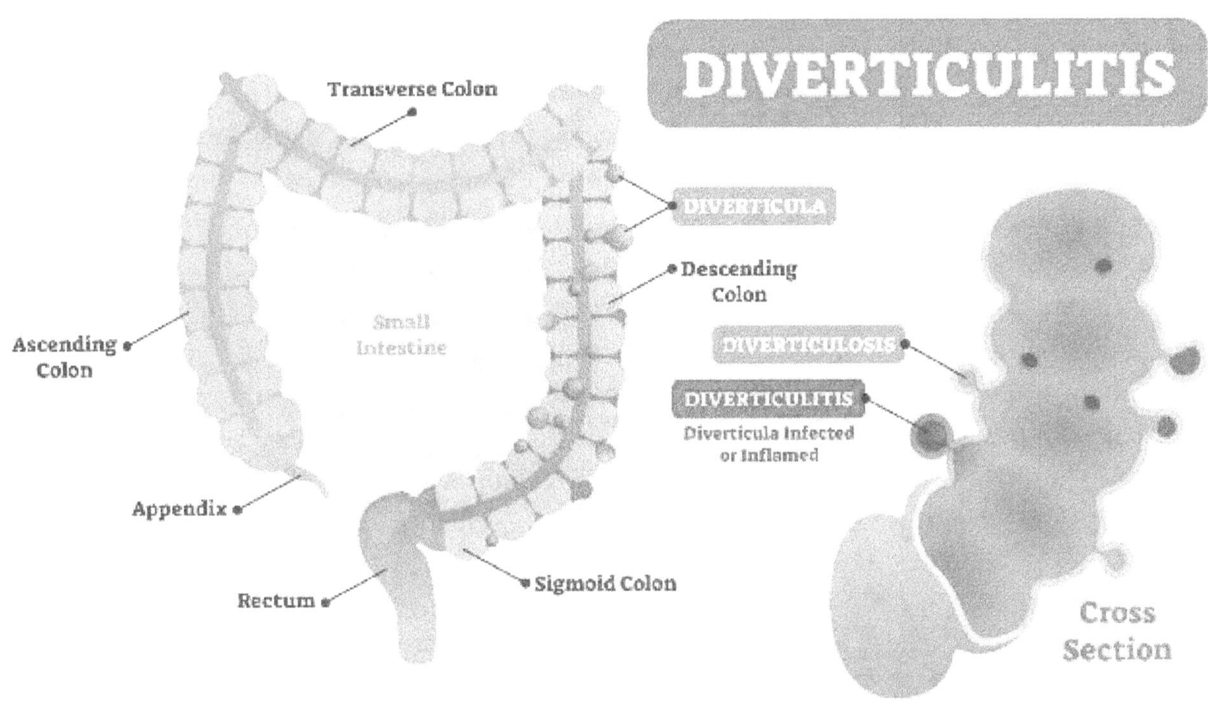

Welcome to a journey through understanding Diverticulitis, a condition that touches the lives of many yet often lurks in the shadows of misunderstanding. Imagine your gut as a garden, where everything usually flourishes in a delicate balance. But sometimes, just as a garden can face unexpected issues, so too can our digestive systems, leading to the development of conditions like diverticulitis.

At its core, diverticulitis occurs when small, bulging pouches, or diverticula, form in the digestive tract. These pouches are common, especially as we age, but the problem arises when they become inflamed or infected. It's akin to having a beautiful path through a garden which suddenly sprouts thorns—an unwelcome obstacle that can cause pain and discomfort.

The causes of this condition are multifaceted, ranging from genetic predispositions to lifestyle factors like diet and exercise. However, one of the key elements often lies in the foods we eat. As we delve into the causes and risk factors associated with diverticulitis, we'll explore how what you ingest plays a pivotal role, not just in the emergence of this condition, but also in its management and prevention.

Managing diverticulitis isn't solely about treating symptoms. It's about embarking on a holistic path that begins with understanding and awareness. Through this understanding, you can become proactive about your dietary choices, transforming your eating habits into powerful tools for health maintenance and symptom prevention.

So, as we move forward in this chapter, remember that learning about diverticulitis is the first step in owning your health journey. With each page, you'll gain not only knowledge but also practical strategies that can lead to lasting relief and a healthier gut. Together, let's cultivate a garden of gut health that thrives and supports your overall wellbeing, allowing you to lead a life full of vitality and comfort.

1.1 What is Diverticulitis?

Diverticulitis may sound complex, but it begins with a basic concept—little pouches, known as diverticula, that form mainly in the lower part of your large intestine. These pouches are not inherently harmful and are, in fact, quite common, especially as we grow older. However, the complications begin when these tiny formed pouches become inflamed or infected, a condition we then call diverticulitis.

Think of your digestive tract as a bustling highway. Over the years, it deals with the wear and tear of what we consume—ranging from highly processed snacks to rich, fibrous vegetables. As the lining of the intestine pushes against the waste that travels along this highway, pressure builds. In some spots, especially weak ones, this pressure can cause little bulges to form, creating diverticula. It's like pushing a finger against the side of a balloon; the pressure causes it to bulge outward. In ideal conditions, these bulges are harmless and unnoticed. But when they become inflamed, your body raises an alarm in the form of diverticulitis.

This inflammation or infection can bring about a sudden and often severe set of symptoms. Patients may experience sharp and persistent pain, typically on the lower left side of the abdomen. This pain could escalate when eating or shortly after meals. Besides pain, other common symptoms include nausea, a significant change in bowel habits (constipation or, less commonly, diarrhea), and fever—an indicator of inflammation and infection in the body.

When such symptoms arise, diagnosing diverticulitis involves a blend of clinical examination and diagnostic tests. Doctors typically start with a detailed discussion about the patient's dietary habits, bowel movements, and overall health history. Medical imaging techniques such as a CT scan are often utilized to confirm the presence of inflamed diverticula and to rule out other potential health issues.

Beyond the clinical, there exists in everyday conversation numerous misconceptions about diverticulitis. One common myth is that seeds and nuts are direct culprits of this condition. For many years, patients were advised to avoid these foods based on the theory that small particles could lodge in the diverticula and initiate inflammation. However, recent research suggests that seeds and nuts do not contribute to this condition and that avoiding them may be unnecessary. Instead, a lack of fiber is a more significant risk factor, as fiber helps keep waste soft and movements regular, preventing the high pressure that can lead to the formation of diverticula.

Also misunderstood is the idea that diverticulitis is solely a disease of the elderly. While risk increases with age, diverticulitis has been observed in younger adults too, especially those who lead sedentary lifestyles or those who consume a diet low in fiber and high in processed foods.

Another significant aspect is distinguishing between diverticulosis and diverticulitis. Diverticulosis refers to the mere presence of diverticula, which, for many individuals, remains symptom-free and harmless throughout their lives. Diverticulitis, in contrast, denotes the phase where inflammation or infection is present, necessitating medical intervention and possible dietary modifications.

Understanding the evolutionary backdrop of our digestive anatomy offers insights into diverticulitis. Our modern diet, drastically different from the fiber-rich fare of our ancestors, imposes less need for extensive digestion, which might contribute to weaker points along our intestinal tract over time. By reconnecting with diets rich in fiber, not only do we pay homage to our ancestral dietary patterns but we also arm our gut with the necessary tools to stay strong and resilient against conditions like diverticulitis.

Knowing the risk factors, too, empowers prevention. Age, an inactive lifestyle, smoking, and the use of certain medications, including steroids and opioids, are well-known risk factors. But with proactive measures such as regular physical activity and a balanced diet rich in vegetables, fruits, and whole grains, the likelihood of developing diverticulitis can be minimized.

Our intestinal health is critically intertwined with our overall well-being, influencing not only our physical comfort but also our mood and energy levels. By fostering awareness and correcting misconceptions, we can take meaningful steps toward not just managing but preventing diverticulitis. This is not merely about avoiding discomfort but about enhancing the quality of life. """); This holistic view transforms the condition from a feared abnormality into another manageable aspect of our health, with knowledge and lifestyle adjustments as keys to both mitigation and solution. In doing so, we don't just treat diverticulitis; we embrace a healthier, more vibrant life.

1.2 Causes and Risk Factors

Understanding the causes and risk factors of diverticulitis is like unraveling a complex web in which lifestyle, diet, genetics, and age all play integral roles. This multifaceted approach helps us to see not just the how, but also the why behind this condition, guiding us toward more effective, proactive management strategies.

Let's begin with age, an uncontested influencing factor in the development of diverticulitis. As we age, the natural strength and elasticity of our gastrointestinal tract diminishes. This degradation makes it easier for diverticula to form when there is increased pressure from the inside, such as when we strain during bowel movements. Hence, diverticulitis is more prevalent in older adults, although it's important to note that its incidence in younger populations is steadily rising. This trend likely reflects changes in lifestyle and dietary habits that are not age discriminatory.

Diet plays a perhaps unsurprisingly crucial role in influencing the risk of developing diverticulitis. Diets low in fiber are particularly implicated. Fiber, which is abundant in fruits, vegetables, and whole grains, helps to keep the intestine working efficiently. Without sufficient fiber, the colon must work harder to push stool through the gastrointestinal tract, increasing the pressure that can lead to the formation of diverticula. When these pouches become inflamed, diverticulitis ensues. The Western diet, heavy in processed foods and low in natural fibers, may explain the rising rates of diverticulitis in industrialized countries.

While dietary fiber intake is important, the type of diet can also influence risk factors. Diets high in red meat and fat have been associated with an increased risk of developing diverticulitis, possibly due to the inflammatory properties of these foods. Conversely, vegetarian diets have been linked to a lower risk, likely due to their higher fiber content and the anti-inflammatory effects of many plant-based foods.

Lifestyle factors can also directly impact gut health and the likelihood of developing diverticulitis. Physical inactivity is a significant risk factor. Regular physical activity helps to stimulate intestinal contractions, reducing the pressure inside the colon and thereby decreasing the likelihood of diverticula formation. Conversely, a sedentary lifestyle, prevalent in many modern societies, can increase the chances of developing diverticula and subsequently diverticulitis.

The influence of genetic factors cannot be understated. Although lifestyle and diet play crucial roles, they don't fully account for why some individuals develop diverticulitis while others do not. Studies suggest that genetics contribute to the structural integrity of the colon wall. Individuals with a family history of diverticulitis are at a higher risk, indicating a possible genetic predisposition to weaker spots in the colon that are more susceptible to diverticula formation.

Beyond these factors, other emerging risk factors include the use of certain medications and tobacco use. Nonsteroidal anti-inflammatory drugs (NSAIDs), steroids, opiates, and even over-the-counter pain relievers like ibuprofen have been linked to increased risk of diverticulitis, likely due to their effects on gut motility and inflammation. Likewise, smoking not only decreases blood flow to the colon, impairing its health and function but also increases the risk of developing complications if diverticulitis occurs.

Even the state of one's microbial health, the microbiome, plays a part. Our gut hosts billions of bacteria, and an imbalance—dysbiosis—can lead to numerous digestive conditions, including potentially diverticulitis. A healthy, fiber-rich diet supports a robust microbiome, which in turn protects the intestinal walls and may prevent the formation of diverticula.

In chronicling these risk factors, the role of awareness becomes clear. By understanding the complex interactions of these variables, individuals can adopt lifestyle changes that drastically reduce their risks. For the elderly, it becomes crucial to maintain an active lifestyle and a diet rich in fibers and low in red meat and refined sugars. For those with a genetic predisposition, this knowledge could lead to earlier and more frequent screenings, potentially catching signs of diverticulitis before it becomes severe. Similarly, anyone on long-term medication should be aware of the associated risks and manage them proactively through diet and lifestyle adjustments.

Ultimately, understanding the causes and risks associated with diverticulitis empowers each of us to take control of our health. It's about making informed choices—embracing a lifestyle that supports our gut health and making adjustments that reflect our personal risk factors and family history. By doing so, we not only address diverticulitis but also enhance our overall health and well-being, reinforcing the idea that a healthy gut is a cornerstone of a vibrant, active life.

1.3 Managing Diverticulitis Through Diet

Navigating diverticulitis often begins at the end of your fork. The journey through dietary management is key to mitigating symptoms and preventing flare-ups. After all, the gut is not only a pathway for food but also an avenue of health and wellness, influencing everything from our mood to our immune system. Understanding the role of diet in managing diverticulitis not only provides relief but also empowers us in the face of this condition.

The cornerstone of diverticulitis management is dietary modification, aimed at reducing inflammation and minimizing the pressure exerted on the colon walls. A fiber-rich diet, often recommended in the remission phase of diverticulitis, aids in this. Fiber contributes to stool bulk and softness, facilitating easier transit through the colon and reducing the risk of the pouches becoming inflamed or infected. Thus, integrating a high-fiber diet is one of the essential steps in managing diverticulitis, especially during periods of remission.

However, during an acute flare-up, the dietary strategy changes significantly. Health professionals typically recommend a low-fiber or clear liquid diet to give the gut a chance to rest and heal. This might include broths, water, and a small selection of juice or tea. Gradually, as inflammation subsides, solid foods are reintroduced, starting from low-fiber options and slowly transitioning back to high-fiber foods.

Identifying safe versus trigger foods is another crucial step for individuals managing diverticulitis. While safe foods generally include well-cooked vegetables, ripe fruits, and lean proteins, trigger foods can vary from person to person. Commonly, these trigger foods include corn, popcorn, and certain nuts and seeds—though, as research evolves, the list of definitive trigger foods is becoming less rigid. More recent findings suggest that these foods might not increase the risk of complications as previously thought.

Besides fiber, focusing on anti-inflammatory foods can profoundly benefit individuals with diverticulitis. Foods rich in omega-3 fatty acids, like fish, flaxseeds, and walnuts, can help reduce inflammation. Turmeric, ginger, and green tea are also known for their anti-inflammatory properties and can be beneficial additions to the diet.

Prebiotics and probiotics play an underrated yet critical role in gut health. They help maintain and restore the balance of gut bacteria, which is vital for overall digestive health and can be particularly beneficial in managing conditions like diverticulitis. Prebiotic foods, such as bananas, onions, and garlic, nourish the good bacteria in the gut, while probiotic foods like yogurt, sauerkraut, and kefir add beneficial bacteria to the digestive system.

Understanding which foods to eat and avoid is one thing, but knowing why can transform a diet plan from a list of commands to a personalized health guide. For instance, during a diverticulitis attack, reducing fiber limits the material that passes through the colon, thereby reducing the workload of the bowel as it heals. Meanwhile, during remission, a high-fiber diet helps prevent the formation of stool that can exert pressure on the walls of the colon and potential weak spots where diverticula might form.

Additionally, the timing of food intake and portion sizes can also influence gut health in the context of diverticulitis. Smaller, more frequent meals are often more manageable on the gut than large, heavy meals, which can exert greater pressure on the colon.

Drinking plenty of fluids is another pivotal aspect of managing diverticulitis. Adequate hydration is crucial as it supports the digestive system, helps dissolve nutrients and fiber, and ensures smooth passage through the intestines which can minimize the risk of diverticulitis flare-ups.

In conclusion, while each person's experience with diverticulitis can be unique, the common denominator often lies in dietary management. Adopting a diet that reduces inflammation, balances gut bacteria, and manages the physical stress on the colon can have a profound effect. These changes can not only help manage the symptoms and prevent flare-ups of diverticulitis but also enhance overall digestive health, which is integral to a vital and vibrant life.

By understanding not just the what but the why behind dietary recommendations for diverticulitis, individuals can tailor their eating habits to better support their colon health, ultimately leading to improved well-being and a more active and enjoyable life. This proactive approach transforms the battle against diverticulitis from one of endurance into one of empowerment, where every meal nourishes not just the body, but also the soul.

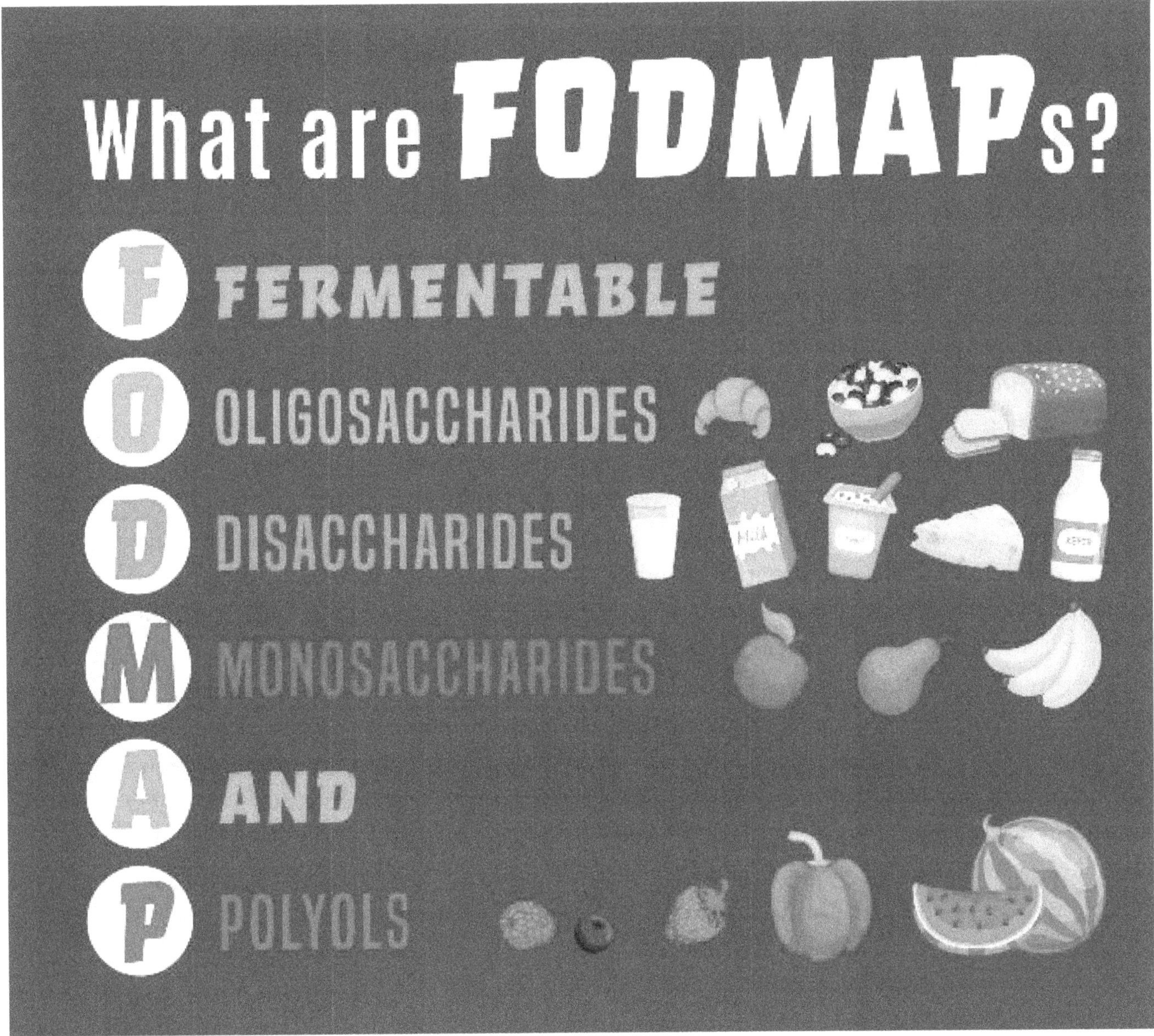

Embarking on a journey to manage diverticulitis through diet isn't just about avoiding certain foods—it's about embracing an entirely new perspective on eating. In this chapter, we will explore the core dietary principles that not only aim to soothe and heal but also revitalize your gut health profoundly.

Understanding the balance and types of food we consume plays a pivotal role in our health. Particularly for those managing diverticulitis, what you put on your plate can mean the difference between a day filled with discomfort and one brimming with vitality. The journey begins with fiber—a key player in digestive health. While the mere mention of fiber often brings to mind images of bland and unappealing foods, let's challenge that notion. Imagine instead a plateful of colorful berries, wholesome grains, and verdant, crispy leafy greens. These foods are not only rich in fiber but also full of flavor and essential nutrients that cater to both your palate and your condition.

Next, we shift our focus to the foods known for their anti-inflammatory properties. Picture the rich, golden hues of turmeric and the vibrant oranges of sweet potatoes. These aren't just pleasing to the eye—they're packed with natural compounds that can calm inflammation in your digestive system, easing the symptoms of diverticulitis.

Lastly, we will tackle the concept of FODMAPs—certain types of carbohydrates that are difficult for some people to digest. Understanding which foods contain these and how to adjust your intake isn't just about following a list; it's about listening to your body and noticing how different foods impact your symptoms.

As we delve into these principles, remember that each meal is an opportunity to not only nourish your body but to ease your symptoms and possibly prevent the recurrence of flare-ups. With each soothing soup, each vibrant salad, and every thoughtful meal, you are taking steps towards a healthier, more comfortable life. This chapter isn't just a set of guidelines—it's a gateway to a new way of eating and living, one that respects and supports your body's needs.

2.1 The Role of Fiber

In the landscape of digestive health, particularly when dealing with conditions like diverticulitis, fiber holds a spotlight, almost revolutionary in its impact yet humble in its presence in everyday foods. Fiber might seem a common thread in dietary discussions, yet its profound impact on our well-being demands a closer look, especially for those navigating the complexities of diverticulitis.

Fiber, broadly categorized into soluble and insoluble forms, serves multiple key functions in managing digestive health. Soluble fiber, which dissolves into a gel-like texture in water, aids in moderating blood glucose levels and lowering cholesterol. Found in oats, nuts, seeds, beans, lentils, and some fruits and vegetables, it plays the role of a soothing agent for the digestive tract. On the other hand, insoluble fiber, found in whole grains, wheat bran, and vegetables, adds bulk to the stool and facilitates its movement through the digestive system, pivotal in preventing the constipation that could exacerbate diverticulitis.

Imagine the journey of food as it travels through the digestive pathway: fiber acts not just as a broom, sweeping through the intestines, but as a caretaker that nurtures and regulates the environment. It's fascinating how something so seemingly inert can be so dynamic in action. For individuals with diverticulitis, the adjustment in fiber intake should be gradual. A sudden increase can lead to discomfort, bloating, or gas. The key is incremental inclusion, allowing the body to adapt, ensuring the intestine works neither too hard nor too little but maintains a balanced pace.

In illustrating the importance of fiber, consider the story of a garden. Just as a variety of plants enriches the soil, a variety of fiber-rich foods enriches your body. Each type of fiber has a different role to play, akin to how some plants might add nutrients while others aerate the soil. In a balanced diet, fiber-rich foods can help create an environment in the gut that is conducive to healing and long-term health, reducing inflammation and supporting the beneficial bacteria residing in our gut microbiome.

Including more fiber in the diet for someone with diverticulitis does not mean overhauling meals but integrating fiber thoughtfully into the diet. Begin with familiar foods that naturally contain fiber, such as adding a variety of beans to a salad or choosing whole grain options instead of refined grains. It's an art of making small switches that collectively assemble a mosaic of nutritious, fiber-dense meals. For those unsure of where to start, beginning with a serving of steamed vegetables at dinner or a piece of fresh fruit as an afternoon snack can be simple, yet effective steps.

However, it is not just about adding fiber to the diet; it's also about how you add it. Drinking plenty of fluids is essential when increasing fiber intake. Water works in tandem with fiber, helping to soften the bulk and promote a smoother journey through the intestines. Consider fiber and water as dance partners in the waltz of digestion, each step calculated and essential for maintaining rhythm and balance.

This approach not only aids direct symptom management but also builds a foundation for long-term digestive health. Engaging regularly with a fiber-rich diet can diminish the likelihood of flare-ups and complications associated with diverticulitis. More so, this proactive dietary management can improve overall quality of life, minimizing fear around food and eating, and restoring confidence in one's dietary choices.

Further punctuating the role of fiber, let us not overlook its preventative capabilities. Regular intake of fiber is linked with a decreased risk of developing diverticulosis in the first place. It suggests not just a treatment but a preventive strategy, underscoring the axiom that often, the best cure is prevention.

So, as we weave through the discussions about dietary fibers, let us not see it merely as a prescription but as a pathway. A pathway that leads to improved digestive health, enhanced well-being, and a renewed sense of control over one's health destiny. Fiber is more than just a dietary component; it's a daily commitment to nurturing your body, understanding its signals, and responding with care.

Harnessing the power of fiber in managing diverticulitis is therefore not just about following medical advice—it's about embarking on a journey of self-awareness and adjustment, responding to the body's needs with a blend of knowledge and compassion. In this journey, each meal enriched with fiber is not just nourishment, but a step towards a vibrant, healthier life.

2.2 Anti-Inflammatory Foods

In the quest to manage and mitigate diverticulitis, understanding the intricate dance of inflammation within our bodies is crucial. It's a phenomenon that often plays a defensive role protecting us from illnesses and repair body tissue. However, when inflammation becomes chronic, it can exacerbate the symptoms of conditions like diverticulitis, leading to discomfort and potential complications. This brings us to the pivotal role of anti-inflammatory foods in our diets, which not only delight our taste buds but also support our bodies' defenses against inflammation.

Imagine your body as a carefully moderated ecosystem, where every element influences the others. In this system, certain foods act like soothing balm, modulating the body's inflammatory responses. These foods are rich in antioxidants, fibers, and omega-3 fatty acids, which collectively contribute to reducing inflammation, thereby aiding those with diverticulitis in easing their symptoms.

Turmeric, for instance, with its vibrant golden color, is not just a staple in culinary traditions around the world; it's a powerhouse of curcumin, a chemical known for its significant anti-inflammatory properties. Picture adding a teaspoon of turmeric to a smoothie or a curry, introducing not just flavor but a burst of anti-inflammatory action to your meal.

Similarly, fatty fish such as salmon, mackerel, and sardines, are abundant in omega-3 fatty acids. These components are stellar at fighting inflammation. These fish do not need elaborate preparations to be beneficial. Grilled with a touch of olive oil, some garlic, and a sprinkle of herbs, they transform into a dish that satisfies the palate while pacifying inflammation within your body.

Green leafy vegetables like spinach, kale, and collards, are loaded with antioxidants that play a role in combating the free radicals which can trigger inflammation. Integrating these greens can be as simple as tossing them into a salad or sautéing them lightly with herbs and high-quality fats like those found in avocado oil.

Speaking of avocados, they themselves are a treasure trove of beneficial compounds, including potassium, magnesium, fiber, and heart-healthy monounsaturated fats. They contribute not just to reducing inflammation but also to overall health vigor, supporting heart health, and providing creamy texture and rich flavor to dishes.

Berries, with their wide varieties including blueberries, strawberries, raspberries, and blackberries, offer high levels of antioxidants known as anthocyanins, which have been researched for their ability to reduce inflammation and contribute to the healthy management of many chronic diseases like diverticulitis. Incorporating berries into your diet can be as delightful as adding them to a morning oatmeal or blending them into a smoothie.

On the other side of these additions are nuts like almonds and walnuts, which contain healthy fats, fibers, and vitamins that are essential in an anti-inflammatory diet. Imagine snacking on a handful of these nuts or garnishing a salad with them to add a crunchy texture and a boost of anti-inflammatory power.

Furthermore, the inclusion of olive oil as a primary fat source stands out for its health benefits, especially extra virgin olive oil, which is high in oleocanthal, an ingredient known for its anti-inflammatory effects. Drizzle it over salad or mix it into vinaigrettes to enrich your meals with its flavors and health benefits.

Each of these foods brings its unique shades to the palette of our diet, painting a picture of vibrant health and proactive disease management. Simple modifications and choices can lead not only to alleviating the symptoms of diverticulitis but also to an enhanced quality of life. Cooking, therefore, does not only preserve nutrients but transforms these ingredients into healing meals. Gentle cooking methods like steaming, poaching, or baking can be particularly beneficial, helping to retain the integrity of nutrients that mitigate inflammation.

Through understanding and utilizing the anti-inflammatory properties of these foods, we also unravel layers of benefits that extend beyond diverticulitis. This isn't just about avoiding discomfort but fostering an environment within your body that is primed for long-term health and vitality. The consumption of anti-inflammatory foods creates a symphony in the body, where each nutrient plays its part in reducing flare-ups and promoting healing.

Thus, embracing a diet rich in anti-inflammatory foods is not merely a recommendation but a lifestyle shift that nurtures your body from the core, ameliorates symptoms, and enhances your overall well-being. This approach to diet creates a foundation not just for managing diverticulitis but for flourishing despite it, proving once again that the power of food extends far beyond the plate.

2.3 Understanding and Managing FODMAPs

Navigating the waters of a diverticulitis-friendly diet introduces us to various dietary considerations—among these, understanding and managing FODMAPs stands crucial. FODMAPs—an acronym for Fermentable Oligosaccharides, Disaccharides, Monosaccharides, and Polyols—are short-chain carbohydrates that are poorly absorbed in the small intestine. For someone with sensitive gastrointestinal issues such as diverticulitis, these can be a major trigger of discomfort and inflammation.

Grasping the role of FODMAPs in your diet is akin to understanding a complex character in a novel. Each type of FODMAP can appear in various chapters of your daily eating habits, impacting your digestive story profoundly. For many, foods high in these carbohydrates can ferment in the gut, leading to the production of gases and attracting water into the colon—both of which can lead to symptoms such as bloating, gas, stomach pain, and altered bowel habits.

Embarking on a low-FODMAP diet often opens a new chapter in managing these symptoms. It begins with identifying and eliminating high-FODMAP foods, then systematically reintroducing them to discern which specific types or quantities are tolerable. It's a process of trial and personalization, meticulously figuring out the optimal dietary balance that supports your digestive health without triggering symptoms.

The common high-FODMAP foods include onions and garlic, which are common culprits in exacerbating symptoms. These form the backbone of flavor in many traditional recipes but can also lead to considerable distress. Additionally, certain fruits like apples, pears, and stone fruits; vegetables such as cauliflowers, mushrooms, and asparagus; dairy products rich in lactose; and wheat and rye products are significant sources of FODMAPs.

However, the path of a low-FODAPM diet isn't merely about avoidance. It includes embracing an array of other nutritious alternatives. For instance, instead of onion and garlic, the diet encourages the use of herbs and spices like chives, basil, and saffron which can deliver flavor without the distress. Fruits like bananas, oranges, and grapes; vegetables such as carrots, cucumbers, and lettuce; lactose-free dairy or dairy alternatives, and grains like oats, quinoa, and rice, pave the way for a gentler but equally enriching culinary journey.

Embarking on this dietary adjustment, consider the narrative of a well-structured regimen, initially stringent, gradually becoming tailored to your personal tolerances. Think of the first phase, the elimination, as setting the stage—removing all high-FODMAP foods to clear the symptoms. This is followed by the critical reintroduction phase, where you reintroduce foods one group at a time, noting how each affects you. This phase is akin to unfolding the nuances of each character—each food—understanding its role in your digestive story. Ultimately, the personalization phase allows you to establish a long-term eating strategy that maintains a broad, nutritional palette while managing your symptoms.

Adherence to a low-FODMAP diet can be markedly eased with proper guidance from nutrition experts who are familiar with the intricacies of such a regimen. Their expertise can help demystify the complexities of FODMAPs, ensuring you're not unnecessarily restricting your diet and still reaping the benefits of a diverse palette of nutrients.

Furthermore, while managing FODMAPs is a cornerstone in the culinary management of diverticulitis, the overarching theme is balance. It's not just about subtracting but about creating a harmonious blend of what can be included to maintain both the joy of eating and the health of your digestive system.

In this journey, the narrative weaves through learning and understanding, not just avoidance. Each meal becomes a deliberate choice contributing to a narrative of well-being, turning each day into an opportunity to support your health without feeling deprived. Managing FODMAPs isn't just a dietary restriction; it's a proactive, informed approach to eating that respects the body's needs and the soul's cravings for nourishing, delicious meals.

Thus, while the road to managing diverticulitis through diet is paved with various strategies, understanding and handling FODMAPs is integral. It encourages not just a symptomatic relief but also a deeper understanding and connection with the foods we eat, transforming our approach to diet from one of restriction to one of mindful, healthful indulgence.

CHAPTER 3: BREAKFAST RECIPES

As dawn breaks, a new day begins, and with it comes the opportunity to nurture your body and soothe your digestive system. Breakfast, often called the most important meal of the more so when managing diverticulitis. It sets the tone for a day of nourishment and can significantly influence your digestive comfort.

In this chapter, we explore a collection of breakfast recipes that are not only quick and soothing but are meticulously crafted to support your gut health and provide a gentle start to your day. Whether you have ample time in the morning or only a few moments before your day begins, these recipes cater to your needs while ensuring that you start your day right, both nutritionally and digestively.

Visualize beginning your day with a warm, soothing bowl of oatmeal infused with a hint of cinnamon and perhaps a drizzle of honey for sweetness. Such meals are not just comforting; they're packed with the right kind of fibre — soluble fibre, which helps in managing the symptoms of diverticulitis by aiding digestion and reducing flare-ups.

For those mornings when time is a whisper, protein-packed smoothies can be a godsend. Imagine blending fresh, anti-inflammatory fruits with a scoop of protein powder and a dash of almond milk. It's a rejuvenating drink that wakes up your senses and your digestive system with minimal effort and maximum taste.

And then, there are days when you may crave something more substantial, something to sit down with and savor. Light and easy egg dishes can be your go-to during such moments. Eggs, versatile and gentle, can be prepared in ways that are both satisfying and light on the gut. Think of a soft-scrambled egg with a side of steamed spinach—simple, yet fulfilling and gentle on a sensitive stomach.

Each recipe in this chapter acts as a stepping stone towards a healthier you, reinforcing the notion that managing diverticulitis doesn't mean sacrificing enjoyable and flavorful meals. It's about rediscovering the joy of eating, knowing that each food choice supports your journey to long-term health and vitality. This chapter promises you that starting your day on the right note could indeed be as delicious as it is healing.

3.1 WARM, SOOTHING CEREALS

GINGER PEAR BARLEY PORRIDGE

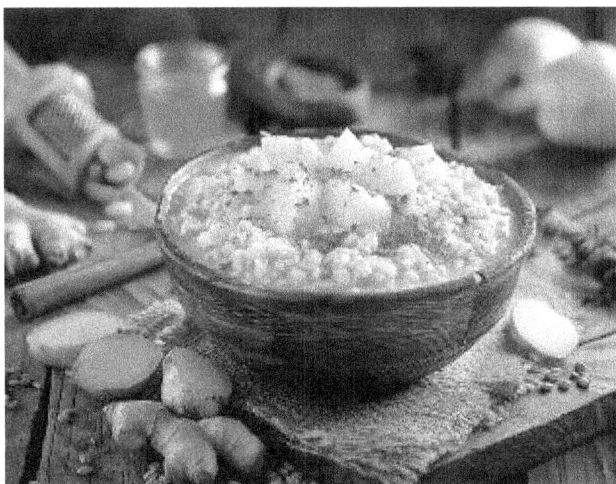

Preparation Time: 10 min
Cooking Time: 25 min
Mode of Cooking: Stovetop
Servings: 2

Ingredients:

- ½ cup pearl barley, rinsed
- 1 large pear, diced
- 1 Tbsp fresh ginger, grated
- 2 cups water
- 1 cup almond milk
- 1 Tbsp honey
- 1/4 tsp cinnamon
- Pinch of salt

Directions:

Combine water, barley, and salt in a medium saucepan and bring to a boil

Reduce heat to low, cover, and simmer for 20 min

Add pear, ginger, honey, and cinnamon

Pour in almond milk and simmer for another 5 min, stirring occasionally

Serve warm

Tips:

- Add a dollop of Greek yogurt for extra creaminess
- Sprinkle with chia seeds for added fiber and nutrients
- Enjoy with a cup of herbal tea for a complete soothing meal

Nutritional Values: Calories: 215, Fat: 1.5g, Carbs: 47g, Protein: 3g, Sugar: 12g, Sodium: 45 mg, Potassium: 240 mg, Cholesterol: 0 mg

Creamy Millet and Pumpkin Cereal

Preparation Time: 15 min
Cooking Time: 30 min
Mode of Cooking: Stovetop
Servings: 4
Ingredients:

- 1 cup millet, thoroughly rinsed
- 2 cups diced pumpkin
- 3 cups water
- 1 cup coconut milk
- 2 Tbsp maple syrup
- ½ tsp ground nutmeg
- ½ tsp ground ginger
- Pinch of salt

Directions:

Toast rinsed millet in a dry pan until slightly golden for about 3 min

Add water and salt, bring to a boil, then add pumpkin

Reduce heat to a simmer, cover, and cook for 25 min

Stir in coconut milk, maple syrup, nutmeg, and ginger

Cook for an additional 5 min

Serve warm

Tips:

- Serve with a sprinkle of toasted pumpkin seeds for a crunchy texture
- Pair with a slice of gluten-free toast for added fiber
- Incorporate a spoonful of flaxseed for an omega-3 boost

Nutritional Values: Calories: 235, Fat: 5g, Carbs: 43g, Protein: 6g, Sugar: 7g, Sodium: 30 mg, Potassium: 250 mg, Cholesterol: 0 mg

Spiced Quinoa Apple Hot Cereal

Preparation Time: 10 min
Cooking Time: 20 min
Mode of Cooking: Stovetop
Servings: 2
Ingredients:

- 1 cup quinoa, rinsed and drained
- 1 large apple, peeled and grated
- 2 cups almond milk
- 1 tsp cinnamon
- ½ tsp nutmeg
- ¼ cup raisins
- 2 Tbsp honey
- Pinch of salt

Directions:

Combine quinoa, almond milk, and salt in a saucepan and bring to a boil

Reduce heat, cover, and simmer for 15 min

Stir in grated apple, cinnamon, nutmeg, raisins, and honey

Simmer for another 5 min until apples are soft

Serve warm

Tips:

- Top with a swirl of almond butter for added richness and protein
- Garnish with a few slices of fresh apple for a refreshing crunch
- For extra sweetness, drizzle with a little extra honey

Nutritional Values: Calories: 290, Fat: 4g, Carbs: 58g, Protein: 8g, Sugar: 22g, Sodium: 40 mg, Potassium: 410 mg, Cholesterol: 0 mg

Soothing Rice Porridge with Dates and Almonds

Preparation Time: 5 min
Cooking Time: 35 min
Mode of Cooking: Stovetop
Servings: 3
Ingredients:

- ½ cup Jasmine rice, rinsed
- 3 cups water
- 1 cup almond milk
- ¼ cup almonds, chopped
- ⅓ cup dates, pitted and chopped
- 1 Tbsp honey
- ½ tsp vanilla extract
- Pinch of salt

Directions:

Boil water in a medium pot and add rice and salt
Reduce heat to low and simmer uncovered for 30 min, stirring occasionally
Add almond milk, almonds, dates, honey, and vanilla extract
Cook for an additional 5 min
Serve warm

Tips:

- Stir in a spoonful of coconut oil before serving for added richness
- Top with a sprinkle of ground cinnamon or cardamom for enhanced flavor
- Enjoy this porridge as a comforting breakfast or a light dinner

Nutritional Values: Calories: 270, Fat: 6g, Carbs: 50g, Protein: 5g, Sugar: 18g, Sodium: 55 mg, Potassium: 295 mg, Cholesterol: 0 mg

Ginger Turmeric Oat Groats

Preparation Time: 5 min.
Cooking Time: 25 min.
Mode of Cooking: Stovetop
Servings: 2
Ingredients:

- 1 cup oat groats, soaked overnight
- 3 cups water
- 1 tsp ground turmeric
- ½ tsp ground ginger
- ⅛ tsp fine sea salt
- 1 Tbsp honey
- 2 Tbsp flaxseed meal
- Optional toppings: sliced banana, a sprinkle of cinnamon

Directions:

Rinse soaked oat groats under cold water
Combine oat groats, water, turmeric, ginger, and sea salt in a medium saucepan and bring to a boil
Reduce heat to low, cover, and simmer for 20-25 min. or until groats are tender
Remove from heat, stir in honey and flaxseed meal
Serve warm with optional toppings

Tips:

- Add a dollop of Greek yogurt for added creaminess and protein
- Stir in a pinch of black pepper to enhance turmeric absorption

Nutritional Values: Calories: 350, Fat: 5g, Carbs: 70g, Protein: 10g, Sugar: 6g, Sodium: 60mg, Potassium: 240mg, Cholesterol: 0mg

3.2 Protein-Packed Smoothies

Banana Almond Flax Smoothie

Preparation Time: 5 min.
Cooking Time: none
Mode of Cooking: Blending
Servings: 2
Ingredients:

- 1 ripe banana
- 2 Tbsp almond butter
- 1 cup unsweetened almond milk
- 2 Tbsp flaxseeds

- 1 scoop vanilla protein powder
- ½ tsp cinnamon

Directions:

Combine banana, almond butter, almond milk, flaxseeds, protein powder, and cinnamon in a blender and blend until smooth

Pour into glasses and serve immediately

Tips:

- Add a pinch of nutmeg for a spicy twist
- Use frozen banana for a thicker texture
- Blend on high for a creamier consistency

Nutritional Values: Calories: 305, Fat: 15g, Carbs: 27g, Protein: 19g, Sugar: 12g, Sodium: 120 mg, Potassium: 450 mg, Cholesterol: 30 mg

SPINACH GINGER DETOX SMOOTHIE

Preparation Time: 7 min.
Cooking Time: none
Mode of Cooking: Blending
Servings: 2
Ingredients:

- 2 cups fresh spinach leaves
- 1 Tbsp fresh ginger, grated
- 1 apple, cored and sliced
- Juice of 1 lemon
- 1 Tbsp chia seeds
- 1½ cups coconut water
- 1 scoop plant-based protein powder

Directions:

Place spinach, ginger, apple, lemon juice, chia seeds, coconut water, and protein powder into a blender

Blend until smooth and creamy

Serve chilled for refreshing taste

Tips:

- Incorporate a sprig of mint for a fresh aroma
- If too thick, adjust consistency with additional coconut water
- Opt for organic produce to minimize toxin intake

Nutritional Values: Calories: 270, Fat: 4g, Carbs: 40g, Protein: 18g, Sugar: 20g, Sodium: 150 mg, Potassium: 700 mg, Cholesterol: 0 mg

BERRY-GUT HEALING SMOOTHIE

Preparation Time: 6 min.
Cooking Time: none
Mode of Cooking: Blending
Servings: 2
Ingredients:

- 1 cup frozen mixed berries (blueberries, raspberries, blackberries)
- 1 cup kefir
- 1 Tbsp honey
- 1 tsp vanilla extract
- 2 Tbsp ground flaxseed
- 1 scoop whey protein isolate
- ½ cup ice

Directions:

Add all ingredients to a blender and blend on high until smooth

Pour into glasses and garnish with a few whole berries on top for presentation

Tips:

- Use Greek yogurt instead of kefir for a thicker texture
- Drizzle with a bit more honey for added sweetness if needed
- Ensure the berries are fully blended for a smooth texture

Nutritional Values: Calories: 280, Fat: 3g, Carbs: 35g, Protein: 25g, Sugar: 28g, Sodium: 110 mg, Potassium: 380 mg, Cholesterol: 45 mg

TROPICAL TURMERIC PROTEIN SMOOTHIE

Preparation Time: 8 min.
Cooking Time: none
Mode of Cooking: Blending
Servings: 2

Ingredients:

- 1 cup pineapple chunks
- 1 banana
- 1 cup light coconut milk
- 1 tsp turmeric powder
- 1 tsp fresh ginger, grated
- 1 Tbsp golden flaxseed meal
- 1 scoop pea protein powder
- Ice as needed

Directions:

Blend pineapple, banana, coconut milk, turmeric, ginger, flaxseed meal, pea protein powder, and ice together until creamy

Serve immediately with a sprinkle of shredded coconut on top

Tips:

- Add a squeeze of lime juice for a zesty kick
- Blend until completely smooth to avoid fibers from pineapple and ginger
- Use frozen banana for extra creaminess

Nutritional Values: Calories: 315, Fat: 8g, Carbs: 40g, Protein: 21g, Sugar: 20g, Sodium: 85 mg, Potassium: 550 mg, Cholesterol: 0 mg

Banana Almond Bliss Smoothie

Preparation Time: 5 min
Cooking Time: none
Mode of Cooking: Blending
Servings: 2
Ingredients:

- 1 ripe banana
- 2 Tbsp almond butter
- 1 cup unsweetened almond milk
- 1 Tbsp chia seeds
- 1 scoop vanilla protein powder
- 1 tsp cinnamon
- Ice cubes as needed

Directions:

Combine banana, almond butter, almond milk, chia seeds, protein powder, cinnamon, and ice cubes in a blender

Blend on high until smooth and creamy

Pour into glasses and serve immediately

Tips:

- Add a pinch of nutmeg for a spicy twist
- Use frozen banana for a thicker consistency
- Top with a few almond slices for added crunch

Nutritional Values: Calories: 250, Fat: 15g, Carbs: 20g, Protein: 8g, Sugar: 10g, Sodium: 180 mg, Potassium: 300 mg, Cholesterol: 0 mg

3.3 Light and Easy Egg Dishes

Zucchini Ribbon & Feta Egg Muffins

Preparation Time: 15 min
Cooking Time: 25 min
Mode of Cooking: Baking
Servings: 6
Ingredients:

- 6 eggs
- 1 cup grated zucchini, water squeezed out
- 1/2 cup crumbled feta cheese
- 1/4 cup diced red bell pepper
- 1/4 cup chopped fresh basil
- 1 clove garlic, minced
- Salt and pepper to taste

Directions:

Preheat oven to 350°F (175°C)

Whisk eggs in a bowl and mix in zucchini, feta, bell pepper, basil, garlic, salt, and pepper

Pour mixture into greased muffin cups, filling each 3/4 full

Bake until muffins are set and tops are slightly golden, about 25 min

Tips:

- Use a paper towel to squeeze out excess moisture from zucchini to avoid soggy muffins

- Customize with your favorite veggies or herbs for variety

Nutritional Values: Calories: 140, Fat: 9g, Carbs: 3g, Protein: 10g, Sugar: 2g, Sodium: 320 mg, Potassium: 230 mg, Cholesterol: 200 mg

SILKY TURMERIC SCRAMBLE

Preparation Time: 5 min
Cooking Time: 15 min
Mode of Cooking: Stovetop
Servings: 2
Ingredients:

- 4 eggs
- 1 Tbsp olive oil
- 1/2 tsp turmeric powder
- 2 Tbsp milk
- Salt and pepper to taste
- 1 Tbsp chopped chives

Directions:

Heat olive oil over medium heat in a non-stick skillet

Whisk eggs, turmeric, milk, salt, and pepper in a bowl

Pour egg mixture into skillet and gently stir with a silicone spatula, allowing large curds to form and cooking until eggs are softly set

Garnish with chives

Tips:

- Incorporate turmeric slowly to achieve an even color distribution
- Serve immediately for best texture and flavor

Nutritional Values: Calories: 190, Fat: 15g, Carbs: 2g, Protein: 12g, Sugar: 1g, Sodium: 220 mg, Potassium: 130 mg, Cholesterol: 370 mg

GARDEN VEGGIE STEAM OMELETTE

Preparation Time: 10 min
Cooking Time: 15 min
Mode of Cooking: Steaming
Servings: 1
Ingredients:

- 2 eggs
- 1/2 cup chopped spinach
- 1/4 cup thinly sliced carrots
- 1/4 cup sliced mushrooms
- 2 Tbsp water
- Salt and pepper to taste
- 1 Tbsp grated Parmesan cheese

Directions:

Whisk eggs, water, salt, and pepper in a bowl

Stir in spinach, carrots, and mushrooms

Pour into a greased heatproof dish, cover with foil, and place in a steamer over boiling water

Steam until eggs are set, about 15 min

Uncover and sprinkle with Parmesan

Tips:

- Ensure water does not touch the bottom of the egg dish in the steamer to prevent waterlogging
- Experiment with various vegetables according to seasonal availability

Nutritional Values: Calories: 150, Fat: 10g, Carbs: 5g, Protein: 12g, Sugar: 3g, Sodium: 340 mg, Potassium: 250 mg, Cholesterol: 370 mg

HERBED EGG CLOUDS

Preparation Time: 10 min
Cooking Time: 5 min
Mode of Cooking: Baking
Servings: 2
Ingredients:

- 4 eggs, separated
- 1/4 cup crumbled goat cheese
- 1 Tbsp chopped fresh thyme
- 1 Tbsp chopped fresh rosemary
- Salt and black pepper to taste

Directions:

Preheat oven to 450°F (232°C)

Whip egg whites until stiff peaks form

Gently fold in goat cheese, thyme, rosemary, salt, and pepper

Spoon into mounds on a parchment-lined baking sheet, making a small well in the center of each for the yolk

Place an egg yolk in each well

Bake until yolks are just set, about 5 min

Tips:

- Avoid over-beating the whites to keep them fluffy
- Serving immediately is crucial as the clouds can deflate quickly

Nutritional Values: Calories: 145, Fat: 10g, Carbs: 1g, Protein: 12g, Sugar: 1g, Sodium: 190 mg, Potassium: 110 mg, Cholesterol: 215 mg

Herbed Chervil Scrambled Eggs

Preparation Time: 5 min
Cooking Time: 10 min
Mode of Cooking: Stovetop
Servings: 2
Ingredients:

- 4 large eggs
- 2 Tbsp low-fat milk
- 1 Tbsp chervil, finely chopped
- 1 Tbsp chives, finely chopped
- 1 tsp olive oil
- Salt to taste
- Freshly ground black pepper to taste

Directions:

Whisk eggs, milk, chervil, and chives together in a bowl until light and frothy

Heat olive oil in a non-stick skillet over medium-low heat

Pour in the egg mixture; let it set slightly before gently stirring with a wooden spoon until eggs are fluffy and just set but remain moist

Tips:

- Serve immediately with whole-grain toast for added fiber
- Avoid overcooking to retain moisture in the eggs
- Season with salt and pepper after cooking to enhance flavors without over-salting

Nutritional Values: Calories: 215, Fat: 15g, Carbs: 2g, Protein: 13g, Sugar: 2g, Sodium: 320 mg, Potassium: 200 mg, Cholesterol: 372 mg

Chapter 4: Lunch Recipes

As we venture into the soothing midday sun, let's pause and consider the pleasures and importance of lunch in our journey toward better gut health. Despite the rush of the day, this meal holds a gentle power, offering a moment to nourish and recalibrate our bodies in the battle against diverticulitis.

Lunch, for many, is an oasis in the hustle of a busy day—a chance to slow down, even if just for a moment, and feed our body what it truly needs to thrive. Understanding this, I've tailored our lunchtime recipes not just to satisfy your hunger but to soothe and heal your digestive system. Imagine sitting down to a bowl of healing soup, its steam carrying the scents of aromatic herbs that promise relief and care to your inflamed intestines. Or, picture a salad that goes beyond the ordinary greens, crafted with anti-inflammatory ingredients, each bite crunching with the promise of health.

In crafting these recipes, I've drawn on old-fashioned wisdom combined with modern nutritional science to create meals that could be prepared swiftly and savored slowly. Take, for example, our digestive-friendly salads—they're not just thrown together but thoughtfully composed with ingredients known to reduce bloating and prevent further irritation to your gut.

Equally, our easy wraps and rolls can transform your idea of what is possible in a diverticulitis-friendly diet. Utilizing grains that are gentle on the gut, paired with lean proteins and an array of veggies, these wraps offer convenience without the compromise, ideal for those days when time is short but the need for good nutrition isn't.

And remember, each recipe here isn't just about managing symptoms; it's about enjoying what you eat. Food is one of life's joys—even when managing a condition like diverticulitis. My hope is that these recipes remind you that a therapeutic diet does not have to be a restrictive one. With each lunch, you are rebuilding your health, one flavorful, soothing meal at a moment. So pull up a seat, take a breath, and prepare to treat yourself to a midday meal that's as nurturing as it is nourishing.

4.1 Healing Soups and Broths

Chicken Bone Broth

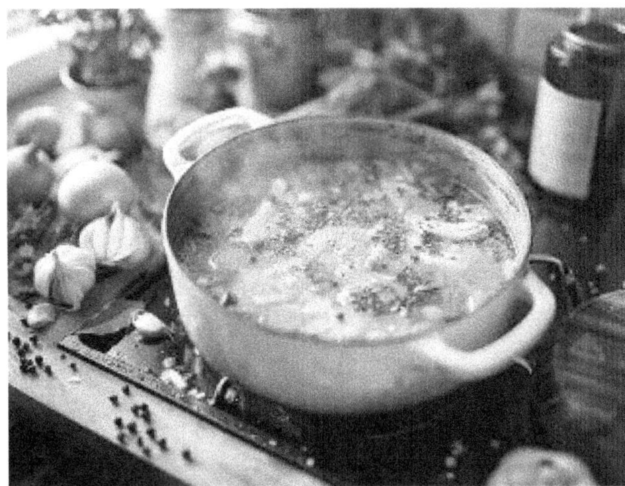

Preparation Time: 10 min
Cooking Time: 3 hr
Mode of Cooking: Stovetop
Servings: 4

Ingredients:

- 2 lb chicken bones
- 1 large onion, quartered
- 2 carrots, chopped
- 3 celery stalks, chopped
- 2 garlic cloves, smashed
- 1 tsp salt
- 1/2 tsp black peppercorns
- 2 bay leaves
- 1 Tbsp apple cider vinegar
- 8 cups water

Directions:

Place chicken bones in a large pot and cover with water

Add onion, carrots, celery, garlic, salt, peppercorns, bay leaves, and apple cider vinegar

Bring to a boil, then reduce to a simmer for 3 hours, skimming foam as necessary

Strain the broth through a fine mesh sieve, discarding solids

Allow to cool before storing in the refrigerator or freezer

Tips:

- Store in glass jars to preserve freshness for up to 5 days in the fridge or 3 months in the freezer
- For a clearer broth, do not stir the pot once the initial ingredients have been added

Nutritional Values: Calories: 40, Fat: 0.5g, Carbs: 2g, Protein: 6g, Sugar: 1g, Sodium: 860 mg, Potassium: 170 mg, Cholesterol: 0 mg

Carrot Ginger Soup

Preparation Time: 15 min
Cooking Time: 30 min
Mode of Cooking: Stovetop
Servings: 4
Ingredients:

- 1 Tbsp olive oil
- 1 lb carrots, peeled and diced
- 1 onion, finely chopped
- 2 Tbsp fresh ginger, grated
- 4 cups vegetable broth
- 1 tsp ground cumin
- 1/2 tsp salt
- 1/4 tsp black pepper
- Fresh cilantro, for garnish

Directions:

Heat olive oil in a large pot over medium heat

Add carrots and onion, sauté until onions are translucent about 5 min

Add ginger, cumin, salt, and pepper, cook for 1 min

Add vegetable broth and bring to a boil

Reduce heat and simmer until carrots are tender, about 25 min

Puree the soup in the pot using an immersion blender until smooth

Tips:

- Garnish with fresh cilantro before serving
- For a creamier texture, add a dollop of coconut milk after blending

Nutritional Values: Calories: 120, Fat: 3g, Carbs: 22g, Protein: 2g, Sugar: 10g, Sodium: 720 mg, Potassium: 550 mg, Cholesterol: 0 mg

Lentil Soup

Preparation Time: 10 min
Cooking Time: 45 min
Mode of Cooking: Stovetop
Servings: 6
Ingredients:

- 1 Tbsp olive oil
- 1 onion, diced
- 2 garlic cloves, minced
- 1 carrot, diced
- 1 celery stalk, diced
- 1 cup dried lentils, rinsed
- 1 tsp ground turmeric
- 1 tsp ground cumin
- 1/2 tsp ground coriander
- 4 cups vegetable stock
- 2 cups water
- Salt and black pepper to taste
- Fresh parsley, chopped for garnish

Directions:

Heat olive oil in a pot over medium heat

Add onion and garlic, sauté until translucent, about 5 min

Add carrot and celery, cook for another 5 min

Add lentils, turmeric, cumin, coriander, vegetable stock, and water

Bring to a boil, then reduce heat and simmer until lentils are tender, about 35 min

Season with salt and pepper to taste

Serve garnished with chopped parsley

Tips:

- Consider soaking lentils overnight to reduce cooking time
- Add a squeeze of lemon juice before serving to enhance flavors

Nutritional Values: Calories: 180, Fat: 3g, Carbs: 30g, Protein: 11g, Sugar: 3g, Sodium: 300 mg, Potassium: 460 mg, Cholesterol: 0 mg

Chicken Bone Broth

Preparation Time: 10 min
Cooking Time: 8 hr
Mode of Cooking: Simmering
Servings: 8
Ingredients:

- 4 lb. of mixed chicken bones
- 1 large onion, quartered
- 2 carrots, chopped
- 3 celery stalks, chopped
- 4 garlic cloves, smashed
- 2 tsp apple cider vinegar
- 10 cups water
- 1 tsp salt
- 1/2 tsp black pepper
- 1 bouquet garni (thyme, bay leaf, parsley)

Directions:

Place bones in a large pot and cover with water; bring to a boil and skim off any foam that forms

Add the onion, carrots, celery, garlic, apple cider vinegar, salt, pepper, and bouquet garni

Reduce heat to a low simmer, cover partially, and cook for 8 hr

Strain broth through a fine-mesh sieve, discarding solids

Tips:

- Add a splash of lemon juice for extra zest and detoxifying properties
- Can be stored in the refrigerator for up to 5 days or frozen for up to 3 months

Nutritional Values: Calories: 40, Fat: 0.5g, Carbs: 1g, Protein: 6g, Sugar: 0.5g, Sodium: 190 mg, Potassium: 170 mg, Cholesterol: 0 mg

Carrot Ginger Soup

Preparation Time: 15 min
Cooking Time: 30 min
Mode of Cooking: Blending & Simmering
Servings: 6
Ingredients:

- 1 Tbsp olive oil
- 1 lb. carrots, peeled and diced
- 2 Tbsp fresh ginger, grated
- 1 medium onion, diced
- 3 cups vegetable broth
- 1 cup coconut milk
- Salt and pepper to taste
- Fresh cilantro for garnish

Directions:

Heat olive oil in a large pot over medium heat

Add onions and sauté until translucent

Add carrots and ginger, cooking for a few minutes more

Pour in vegetable broth and bring to a boil, then reduce to simmer for 25 min

Remove from heat and blend with an immersion blender until smooth

Stir in coconut milk, season with salt and pepper, and heat through

Tips:

- Serve topped with fresh cilantro
- For a creamier texture, use full-fat coconut milk
- Ginger enhances anti-inflammatory benefits

Nutritional Values: Calories: 140, Fat: 9g, Carbs: 13g, Protein: 2g, Sugar: 5g, Sodium: 480 mg, Potassium: 360 mg, Cholesterol: 0 mg

4.2 Digestive-Friendly Salads

Quinoa and Avocado Garden Salad

Preparation Time: 15 min
Cooking Time: none
Mode of Cooking: No Cooking
Servings: 4
Ingredients:

- 1 cup quinoa, rinsed
- 2 cups water
- 1 ripe avocado, cubed
- 1 small cucumber, diced
- 1 red bell pepper, diced
- 1/4 cup fresh parsley, chopped
- 1/4 cup lime juice
- 2 Tbsp extra virgin olive oil
- 1 clove garlic, minced
- Salt and pepper to taste

Directions:

Cook quinoa in water until fluffy, let cool

In a large bowl, combine cooled quinoa, avocado, cucumber, bell pepper, and parsley

In a small bowl, whisk together lime juice, olive oil, and garlic

Pour dressing over salad, toss gently to coat

Season with salt and pepper

Tips:

- Serve immediately or chill to enhance flavors
- Can be stored in the refrigerator for up to 2 days

Nutritional Values: Calories: 248, Fat: 14g, Carbs: 27g, Protein: 5g, Sugar: 3g, Sodium: 13 mg, Potassium: 412 mg, Cholesterol: 0 mg

Beet and Feta Sunshine Salad

Preparation Time: 10 min
Cooking Time: 45 min
Mode of Cooking: Roasting and Mixing
Servings: 4
Ingredients:

- 4 medium beets, trimmed and scrubbed
- 1/2 cup feta cheese, crumbled
- 2 Tbsp sunflower seeds
- 1/4 cup orange juice
- 1 Tbsp olive oil
- 1 Tbsp red wine vinegar
- 1 tsp honey
- Fresh mint leaves, chopped
- Salt and pepper to taste

Directions:

Roast beets at 400°F (204°C) until tender, about 45 min, cool, peel and dice

Combine diced beets, feta cheese, and sunflower seeds in a bowl

In another bowl, whisk together orange juice, olive oil, red wine vinegar, and honey

Drizzle dressing over beet mixture, toss to combine

Garnish with mint, season with salt and pepper

Tips:

- Perfect as a make-ahead salad, flavors meld beautifully overnight
- Roasting beets brings out their natural sweetness

Nutritional Values: Calories: 180, Fat: 9g, Carbs: 20g, Protein: 5g, Sugar: 15g, Sodium: 270 mg, Potassium: 360 mg, Cholesterol: 25 mg

Spinach and Blueberry Vitality Salad

Preparation Time: 10 min
Cooking Time: none
Mode of Cooking: Mixing
Servings: 4
Ingredients:

- 2 cups fresh spinach
- 1 cup blueberries
- 1/4 cup walnuts, toasted
- 1/4 cup goat cheese, crumbled
- 1/4 cup balsamic vinegar
- 1 Tbsp honey

- 1 Tbsp olive oil
- 1 Tbsp chia seeds
- Salt and pepper to taste

Directions:

In a large salad bowl, combine spinach, blueberries, walnuts, and goat cheese

In a small bowl, whisk together balsamic vinegar, honey, and olive oil

Pour dressing over salad, toss to coat evenly

Sprinkle with chia seeds, season with salt and pepper

Tips:

- Enhance with a sprinkle of flax seeds for extra nutrition
- Can be served as a refreshing starter or a light main dish

Nutritional Values: Calories: 207, Fat: 15g, Carbs: 16g, Protein: 6g, Sugar: 10g, Sodium: 125 mg, Potassium: 233 mg, Cholesterol: 13 mg

Quinoa and Avocado Salad with Citrus Vinaigrette

Preparation Time: 15 min
Cooking Time: none
Mode of Cooking: No Cooking
Servings: 4
Ingredients:

- 1 C. quinoa, cooked and cooled
- 1 large avocado, diced
- 1 small red onion, finely chopped
- 1 C. cherry tomatoes, halved
- 1 large cucumber, peeled and diced
- 1/4 C. fresh cilantro, chopped
- for dressing: 2 Tbsp olive oil
- juice of 1 lemon
- juice of 1 lime
- 1 tsp honey
- salt and pepper to taste

Directions:

Combine quinoa, avocado, red onion, cherry tomatoes, cucumber, and cilantro in a large bowl

In a small bowl, whisk together olive oil, juice of lemon and lime, honey, salt, and pepper until emulsified

Pour the dressing over the salad and toss gently until all components are evenly coated

Tips:

- Serve immediately or chill to enhance the flavors
- Customize the dressing by adding a touch of orange zest or a sprinkle of cumin for a different twist
- This salad can be stored in an airtight container in the refrigerator for up to two days

Nutritional Values: Calories: 215, Fat: 14g, Carbs: 20g, Protein: 4g, Sugar: 3g, Sodium: 30 mg, Potassium: 450 mg, Cholesterol: 0 mg

Earthy Beet and Feta Salad with Walnut Dressing

Preparation Time: 20 min
Cooking Time: none
Mode of Cooking: No Cooking
Servings: 4
Ingredients:

- 2 large beets, cooked, peeled and cubed
- 1/2 C. crumbled feta cheese
- 1/4 C. walnuts, toasted and chopped
- 2 Tbsp fresh parsley, finely chopped
- for dressing: 3 Tbsp walnut oil
- 1 Tbsp apple cider vinegar
- 1 tsp mustard
- 1 tsp honey
- salt and pepper to taste

Directions:

Combine beets, feta cheese, walnuts, and parsley in a salad bowl

For the dressing, whisk together walnut oil, apple cider vinegar, mustard, honey, salt, and pepper in a separate bowl until well blended

Pour dressing over beet mixture and toss gently to combine

Tips:

- This salad pairs wonderfully with grilled chicken or fish for a hearty meal
- The feta can be substituted with goat cheese for a creamier texture
- Add a handful of arugula or baby spinach for extra greens

Nutritional Values: Calories: 180, Fat: 12g, Carbs: 15g, Protein: 4g, Sugar: 12g, Sodium: 220 mg, Potassium: 300 mg, Cholesterol: 15 mg

4.3 Easy Wraps and Rolls

Turkey and Spinach Wrap

Preparation Time: 15 min
Cooking Time: none
Mode of Cooking: No Cooking
Servings: 2
Ingredients:

- 2 whole wheat tortillas
- 4 oz. turkey breast, thinly sliced
- 1 cup baby spinach, fresh
- 2 Tbsp low-fat cream cheese, softened
- 1/4 red onion, thinly sliced
- 1/2 avocado, sliced
- 1 tsp lemon juice
- Salt and pepper to taste

Directions:

Spread cream cheese evenly on each tortilla
Lay out turkey slices on top
Add a layer of spinach and red onion slices
In a small bowl, toss avocado slices in lemon juice, then place on top of spinach
Season with salt and pepper
Roll each tortilla tightly, cut in half diagonally

Tips:

- Use a damp paper towel to keep tortillas pliable while assembling
- For a gluten-free option, substitute whole wheat tortillas with gluten-free tortillas

Nutritional Values: Calories: 320, Fat: 15g, Carbs: 27g, Protein: 20g, Sugar: 3g, Sodium: 620 mg, Potassium: 450 mg, Cholesterol: 35 mg

Salmon and Cucumber Rolls

Preparation Time: 20 min
Cooking Time: none
Mode of Cooking: No Cooking
Servings: 2
Ingredients:

- 4 oz. smoked salmon, thinly sliced
- 1 large cucumber, julienned
- 1/4 cup cream cheese, softened
- 1 Tbsp chives, chopped
- 2 tsp dill, fresh, chopped
- 1 Tbsp capers, drained
- Salt and pepper to taste

Directions:

Spread cream cheese on a piece of plastic wrap
Place salmon slices over the cream cheese
Sprinkle chives, dill, and capers evenly over salmon
Arrange julienned cucumber at one end and start rolling tightly using the plastic wrap as a guide
Once rolled, chill for 10 min before slicing into pieces

Tips:

- Serve with a side of light soy sauce or a squeeze of lemon for extra flavor
- Keep rolls refrigerated until serving to maintain firmness

Nutritional Values: Calories: 175, Fat: 9g, Carbs: 5g, Protein: 20g, Sugar: 2g, Sodium: 660 mg, Potassium: 360 mg, Cholesterol: 30 mg

Veggie and Hummus Wrap

Preparation Time: 10 min
Cooking Time: none
Mode of Cooking: No Cooking
Servings: 2

Ingredients:

- 2 spinach tortillas
- 1/2 cup hummus
- 1 carrot, grated
- 1 small beet, grated
- 1/4 cup red cabbage, shredded
- 1/2 bell pepper, thinly sliced
- 1/4 cup alfalfa sprouts
- Salt and pepper to taste

Directions:

Spread hummus evenly over each tortilla

Layer grated carrot, beet, and shredded cabbage on top

Add bell pepper slices and alfalfa sprouts

Season with salt and pepper

Roll tightly, slice in half before serving

Tips:

- To keep vegetables crisp, add them just before serving
- Use different flavored hummus like roasted red pepper for a twist in taste

Nutritional Values: Calories: 290, Fat: 9g, Carbs: 45g, Protein: 9g, Sugar: 5g, Sodium: 390 mg, Potassium: 410 mg, Cholesterol: 0 mg

Chicken Caesar Lettuce Rolls

Preparation Time: 20 min
Cooking Time: none
Mode of Cooking: No Cooking
Servings: 2
Ingredients:

- 6 large lettuce leaves, preferably Romaine
- 6 oz. chicken breast, cooked and shredded
- 2 Tbsp Caesar dressing, low-fat
- 1/4 cup Parmesan cheese, shaved
- 1 tsp Worcestershire sauce
- 1/2 tsp black pepper
- 1 Tbsp lemon juice
- 1/4 cup croutons, whole grain, crushed

Directions:

In a bowl, mix shredded chicken with Caesar dressing, Worcestershire sauce, lemon juice, and black pepper

Lay out lettuce leaves and distribute chicken mixture evenly among them

Sprinkle with Parmesan cheese and add crushed croutons

Roll each lettuce leaf securely, serve immediately

Tips:

- Create a wrap station at the dining table to allow family members to make their own wraps
- For an extra crunch, add freshly toasted croutons just before serving

Nutritional Values: Calories: 214, Fat: 9g, Carbs: 7g, Protein: 24g, Sugar: 1g, Sodium: 450 mg, Potassium: 300 mg, Cholesterol: 50 mg

Turkey and Spinach Wrap

Preparation Time: 15 min
Cooking Time: none
Mode of Cooking: No Cooking
Servings: 2
Ingredients:

- 4 whole wheat tortillas
- 8 oz. thinly sliced turkey breast
- 1 cup baby spinach, washed and dried
- 1 large ripe avocado, sliced
- 1/4 cup low-fat Greek yogurt
- 2 tsp Dijon mustard
- 1/2 tsp garlic powder
- Salt and pepper to taste

Directions:

Spread each tortilla with Greek yogurt

Layer with Dijon mustard

Add slices of turkey breast evenly across the tortilla

Top with avocado slices and a handful of baby spinach

Season with garlic powder, salt, and pepper

Roll the tortillas tightly securing the contents inside

Cut in half diagonally and serve immediately

Tips:

- Opt for a whole grain tortilla for added fiber
- Avocado provides healthy fats that can help with inflammation reduction
- Yogurt can be substituted with a dairy-free alternative for those with lactose intolerance

Nutritional Values: Calories: 320, Fat: 12g, Carbs: 34g, Protein: 20g, Sugar: 2g, Sodium: 600 mg, Potassium: 450 mg, Cholesterol: 30 mg

Chapter 5: Dinner Recipes

As the sun dips below the horizon and the day's hustle winds down, the evening meal becomes not just a necessity but a comforting ritual. Dinner, with its warming, nurturing qualities, is ideally a time when we can not only nourish our bodies but also bring balance and healing, particularly when managing a condition like diverticulitis. In this chapter, our focus shifts to crafting dinner recipes that are both soothing to your gut and appealing to the palate, ensuring that every meal feels like a gentle embrace to your digestive system.

Imagine settling down to a quiet table, with dishes laid out that speak of care and understanding of your digestive needs. The recipes here aren't just food; they're a form of therapy. Each recipe is meticulously designed—tender proteins easy on the digestion, casseroles that bring back the joy of comfort food without the discomfort that usually follows, and slow-cooked dishes that marry convenience with the deep, developed flavors that only time can craft.

The emphasis in these dishes is on simplicity and gentleness, avoiding ingredients known to trigger flare-ups in diverticulitis sufferers. Instead, healing herbs, spices, and cooking methods that enhance digestibility without sacrificing flavor are chosen with care. For instance, a slow-simmered stew with lean cuts of meat and a rich, aromatic broth can be both a salve for the gut and a celebration on the taste buds.

By introducing comforting casseroles and slow-cooked goodness into your dinner plans, you're not just eating to avoid discomfort; you're also breaking the monotony that often shadows a therapeutic diet. These meals promise to restore not just bodily health but also a zest for dining, bringing back the joy of a shared meal with family or the quiet appreciation of a well-prepared dish on a calm evening.

The recipes in this chapter are your allies. They adhere to the principle that even within the boundaries of a diet tailored for digestive health, there can and should be a bounty of flavors and textures to enjoy—proof that food can be both medicine and a source of pleasure.

5.1 Tender and Lean Proteins

Baked Lemon Herb Chicken

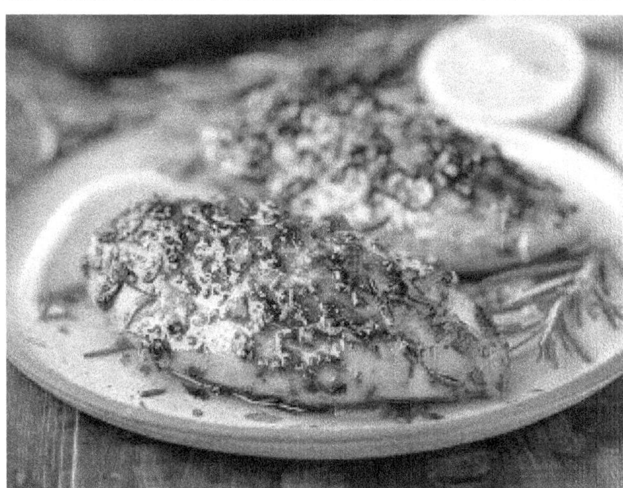

Preparation Time: 10 min
Cooking Time: 30 min
Mode of Cooking: Baking
Servings: 4

Ingredients:

- 4 boneless, skinless chicken breasts
- 2 Tbsp olive oil
- 1 Tbsp fresh rosemary, chopped
- 2 tsp fresh thyme, chopped
- 1 lemon, juiced and zested
- 3 garlic cloves, minced
- Salt to taste
- Black pepper to taste

Directions:

1. Preheat oven to 375°F (190°C)
2. Pat chicken breasts dry and place in a baking dish
3. In a bowl, mix olive oil, rosemary, thyme, lemon juice and zest, garlic, salt, and pepper

4. Pour the mixture over the chicken, ensuring each piece is well coated
5. Bake for 30 min or until chicken reaches an internal temperature of 165°F (74°C)

Tips:

- Let chicken rest for 5 min before serving to retain juices
- Use fresh herbs for a more vibrant flavor
- Pair with a side of steamed vegetables for a complete meal

Nutritional Values: Calories: 210, Fat: 10g, Carbs: 2g, Protein: 27g, Sugar: 1g, Sodium: 70 mg, Potassium: 220 mg, Cholesterol: 70 mg

Steamed Garlic Ginger Fish

Preparation Time: 15 min
Cooking Time: 20 min
Mode of Cooking: Steaming
Servings: 4
Ingredients:

- 4 fish fillets, such as cod or tilapia
- 2 Tbsp ginger, finely grated
- 4 garlic cloves, minced
- 2 Tbsp soy sauce, low sodium
- 1 Tbsp sesame oil
- 1 scallion, thinly sliced
- 1 carrot, julienned
- Salt to taste
- Black pepper to taste

Directions:

1. Fill your steamer with water and bring to a simmer
2. Season the fish fillets with salt and pepper
3. Mix ginger, garlic, soy sauce, and sesame oil in a small bowl
4. Place each fillet on a piece of parchment in the steamer basket
5. Top each with equal parts of the ginger garlic mixture and sprinkle with julienned carrots
6. Steam for about 20 min or until fish flakes easily with a fork

Tips:

- Garnish with scallions before serving
- Serve with a splash of fresh lime juice for extra zest
- Ideal with fluffy jasmine rice

Nutritional Values: Calories: 180, Fat: 5g, Carbs: 3g, Protein: 28g, Sugar: 1g, Sodium: 300 mg, Potassium: 450 mg, Cholesterol: 60 mg

Cumin-Spiced Turkey Patties

Preparation Time: 20 min
Cooking Time: 10 min
Mode of Cooking: Grilling
Servings: 6
Ingredients:

- 1 lb ground turkey
- 1 Tbsp ground cumin
- 2 tsp smoked paprika
- 1 medium red onion, finely chopped
- 2 Tbsp cilantro, chopped
- 1 egg, beaten
- Salt to taste
- Black pepper to taste

Directions:

1. In a large bowl, combine ground turkey, cumin, smoked paprika, red onion, cilantro, and egg
2. Season with salt and pepper and mix until well combined
3. Form into six patties
4. Grill over medium heat for about 5 min on each side or until fully cooked and juices run clear

Tips:

- Serve with a yogurt-based sauce for added moisture
- Pair with a cucumber salad for a refreshing side

- Ensure not to overcook to maintain juiciness of the patties

Nutritional Values: Calories: 170, Fat: 9g, Carbs: 2g, Protein: 20g, Sugar: 1g, Sodium: 85 mg, Potassium: 250 mg, Cholesterol: 80 mg

Lemongrass Infused Grilled Shrimp

Preparation Time: 15 min
Cooking Time: 8 min
Mode of Cooking: Grilling
Servings: 4
Ingredients:

- 1 lb shrimp, peeled and deveined
- 2 stalks lemongrass, outer layers removed and finely minced
- 2 Tbsp coconut oil
- 1 lime, juiced
- 1 Tbsp fish sauce
- 1 tsp chili flakes
- Salt to taste
- Black pepper to taste

Directions:

1. Preheat grill to medium-high
2. In a bowl, combine minced lemongrass, coconut oil, lime juice, fish sauce, and chili flakes
3. Add shrimp and toss to coat evenly
4. Season with salt and pepper
5. Grill shrimp for about 4 min on each side or until opaque and cooked through

Tips:

- Serve immediately with extra lime wedges on the side for added citrus flavor
- Can be enjoyed atop a bed of cilantro-lime rice
- Add grilled vegetables like bell peppers or zucchini for a complete meal

Nutritional Values: Calories: 160, Fat: 8g, Carbs: 3g, Protein: 20g, Sugar: 1g, Sodium: 870 mg, Potassium: 180 mg, Cholesterol: 160 mg

Herb-Crusted Baked Chicken Breast

Preparation Time: 15 min
Cooking Time: 25 min
Mode of Cooking: Baking
Servings: 4
Ingredients:

- 2 lb. chicken breast, boneless and skinless
- 2 Tbsp olive oil
- 1 Tbsp fresh thyme, chopped
- 1 Tbsp fresh rosemary, chopped
- 1 Tbsp fresh parsley, chopped
- 2 cloves garlic, minced
- Salt to taste
- Freshly ground black pepper to taste

Directions:

1. Preheat oven to 375°F (190°C)
2. Pat chicken breasts dry with paper towels
3. Mix oil, thyme, rosemary, parsley, and garlic in a bowl
4. Rub the herb mixture on chicken breasts ensuring they are well coated
5. Season with salt and pepper
6. Place chicken in a baking dish
7. Bake for 25 min or until the internal temperature reaches 165°F (74°C)

Tips:

- Rest chicken before slicing to retain juices
- Serve with steamed vegetables for a complete meal

Nutritional Values: Calories: 310, Fat: 13g, Carbs: 1g, Protein: 46g, Sugar: 0g, Sodium: 95 mg, Potassium: 410 mg, Cholesterol: 120 mg

5.2 Comforting Casseroles

Golden Turmeric Chicken and Rice Casserole

Preparation Time: 15 min.
Cooking Time: 45 min.
Mode of Cooking: Baking

Servings: 6

Ingredients:

- 2 cups brown rice, cooked
- 1 lb. chicken breast, diced
- 1 large onion, finely chopped
- 2 cloves garlic, minced
- 1 Tbsp olive oil
- 1 tsp turmeric powder
- 1/2 tsp ground ginger
- 2 cups low-sodium chicken broth
- 1 cup coconut milk
- 1/2 cup peas
- 1/4 cup chopped cilantro
- Salt and pepper to taste

Directions:

1. Preheat oven to 375°F (190°C)
2. In a skillet, sauté onion and garlic in olive oil until translucent
3. Add diced chicken, turmeric, and ginger, cook until chicken is golden
4. In a casserole dish, combine cooked rice, chicken mixture, peas, chicken broth, and coconut milk
5. Bake covered for 30 min., then uncover and bake for additional 15 min. until crispy on top

Tips:

- Avoid using high heat while sautéing onions to retain subtle flavors
- Garnish with fresh cilantro before serving to enhance the fresh aroma
- Serve hot for better texture and taste

Nutritional Values: Calories: 310, Fat: 9g, Carbs: 35g, Protein: 20g, Sugar: 2g, Sodium: 70 mg, Potassium: 300 mg, Cholesterol: 55 mg

Hearty Vegetable Lasagna

Preparation Time: 20 min.

Cooking Time: 55 min.

Mode of Cooking: Baking

Servings: 8

Ingredients:

- 9 lasagna noodles, pre-cooked
- 1 zucchini, sliced
- 1 bell pepper, chopped
- 1 eggplant, cubed
- 3 cups spinach, fresh
- 2 cups ricotta cheese
- 1 egg
- 2 cups marinara sauce, low-sodium
- 1 cup mozzarella cheese, shredded
- 2 Tbsp Parmesan cheese, grated
- 1 tsp oregano, dried
- Salt and pepper to taste

Directions:

1. Preheat oven to 375°F (190°C)
2. Layer a baking dish with sauce, then noodles, vegetables mixed with ricotta and egg, and sprinkle with mozzarella and Parmesan, repeat until all ingredients are used
3. Cover with foil and bake for 40 min., uncover and bake for additional 15 min. until cheese is bubbly and golden

Tips:

- Use fresh vegetables for a crispier texture
- Let it rest for 10 mins before slicing to solidify layers
- Pair with a side of garlic bread for a full meal

Nutritional Values: Calories: 320, Fat: 12g, Carbs: 35g, Protein: 18g, Sugar: 5g, Sodium: 210 mg, Potassium: 410 mg, Cholesterol: 40 mg

Lentil and Quinoa Bake

Preparation Time: 10 min.

Cooking Time: 50 min.

Mode of Cooking: Baking

Servings: 5

Ingredients:

- 1 cup quinoa, rinsed
- 1 cup brown lentils, rinsed and drained
- 1 carrot, finely chopped
- 1 celery stalk, finely chopped
- 1 onion, minced
- 2 garlic cloves, minced
- 3 cups vegetable broth
- 1 tsp cumin powder
- 1/2 tsp chili flakes
- 2 Tbsp olive oil
- Salt and pepper to taste

Directions:

1. Preheat oven to 375°F (190°C)
2. In a saucepan, heat olive oil and sauté onions, garlic, carrot, and celery until soft
3. Add lentils, quinoa, cumin, chili flakes, and vegetable broth, bring to a boil
4. Transfer to a baking dish, cover with foil, and bake for 40 min., uncover for the last 10 min. to get a crusty top

Tips:

- Stir the mixture halfway through baking to ensure even cooking
- Serve with a dollop of Greek yogurt for creaminess
- Add a squeeze of lemon for a fresh kick before serving

Nutritional Values: Calories: 280, Fat: 6g, Carbs: 40g, Protein: 14g, Sugar: 3g, Sodium: 30 mg, Potassium: 790 mg, Cholesterol: 0 mg

Soothing Chicken and Wild Rice Casserole

Preparation Time: 20 min
Cooking Time: 1 hr
Mode of Cooking: Baking
Servings: 6
Ingredients:

- 2 cups cooked wild rice
- 1 lb cooked chicken breast, shredded
- 1 cup carrots, diced
- 1 cup celery, diced
- 1 medium onion, finely chopped
- 2 cloves garlic, minced
- 2 cups chicken broth, low sodium
- 1 cup plain Greek yogurt
- 2 Tbsp olive oil
- 1 tsp dried thyme
- 1 tsp dried parsley
- Salt and pepper to taste

Directions:

1. Preheat oven to 375°F (190°C)
2. Heat olive oil in a skillet over medium heat and sauté onion, garlic, carrots, and celery until soft
3. Add cooked chicken, rice, thyme, parsley, salt, and pepper, stir to combine
4. Remove from heat and mix in Greek yogurt and chicken broth until well combined
5. Transfer to a baking dish and bake for 45 min

Tips:

- Use Greek yogurt for a creamy texture without added fats
- Opt for low-sodium broth to control the salt content
- Garnish with fresh parsley for enhanced flavor and a touch of color

Nutritional Values: Calories: 310, Fat: 9g, Carbs: 28g, Protein: 26g, Sugar: 4g, Sodium: 180 mg, Potassium: 450 mg, Cholesterol: 55 mg

Hearty Vegetable Lasagna

Preparation Time: 30 min
Cooking Time: 45 min
Mode of Cooking: Baking
Servings: 8
Ingredients:

- 9 lasagna noodles, cooked

- 2 cups spinach, chopped
- 1 cup zucchini, sliced
- 1 cup bell peppers, mixed colors, sliced
- 1 cup ricotta cheese
- 2 cups marinara sauce, low sodium
- 1 cup mozzarella cheese, shredded
- 1 cup mushrooms, sliced
- 2 Tbsp olive oil
- 1 tsp Italian seasoning
- Salt and pepper to taste

Directions:

1. Preheat oven to 375°F (190°C)
2. In a pan, heat olive oil and sauté mushrooms, zucchini, bell peppers, and spinach with salt, pepper, and Italian seasoning until tender
3. Layer bottom of a well-greased baking dish with 3 lasagna noodles
4. Spread half of the vegetable mix, half of the ricotta cheese, and a third of the marinara sauce
5. Repeat layers and finish with remaining noodles, marinara, and top with mozzarella cheese
6. Bake for 30 min

Tips:

- Choose part-skim ricotta and mozzarella to lower fat content without sacrificing taste
- Serve with a side salad for a balanced meal
- Allow the lasagna to rest for 10 min before serving for easier slicing

Nutritional Values: Calories: 275, Fat: 12g, Carbs: 31g, Protein: 14g, Sugar: 5g, Sodium: 210 mg, Potassium: 370 mg, Cholesterol: 30 mg

5.3 Slow-Cooked Goodness

Savory Slow-Cooker Pot Roast

Preparation Time: 15 min
Cooking Time: 8 hr
Mode of Cooking: Slow Cooking
Servings: 6

Ingredients:

- 3 lb. chuck roast
- 1 Tbsp olive oil
- 2 large onions, sliced
- 4 cloves garlic, minced
- 2 cups beef broth
- 1 Tbsp Worcestershire sauce
- 2 Tbsp tomato paste
- 4 carrots, peeled and chopped
- 3 celery stalks, chopped
- 2 large potatoes, peeled and cubed
- 1 tsp dried thyme
- 1 tsp dried rosemary

Directions:

1. Season the chuck roast with salt and pepper and brown in a skillet with olive oil over high heat until all sides are caramelized
2. Place sliced onions and minced garlic in the bottom of the slow cooker
3. Add the browned roast on top
4. Mix beef broth, Worcestershire sauce, and tomato paste together and pour over the roast
5. Arrange the chopped carrots, celery, potatoes around the roast
6. Sprinkle with thyme and rosemary
7. Cover and cook on low for 8 hr

Tips:

- To thicken the gravy, remove 1 cup of the liquid after cooking and whisk with 2 Tbsp of cornstarch, then stir back into the pot
- Let the roast rest for 10 min before slicing
- Serve with the vegetables and drizzle with the cooking juices

Nutritional Values: Calories: 510, Fat: 34g, Carbs: 20g, Protein: 35g, Sugar: 5g, Sodium: 790 mg, Potassium: 1200 mg, Cholesterol: 130 mg

Root Vegetable Slow Cooker Stew

Preparation Time: 20 min
Cooking Time: 6 hr
Mode of Cooking: Slow Cooking
Servings: 5
Ingredients:

- 1 lb. sweet potatoes, cubed
- 1 lb. parsnips, peeled and chopped
- 1 lb. turnips, peeled and chopped
- 2 leeks, cleaned and sliced
- 3 cups vegetable broth
- 1 cup diced tomatoes
- 1 Tbsp apple cider vinegar
- 2 tsp smoked paprika
- 1 sprig rosemary
- Salt and pepper to taste
- 2 tsp olive oil

Directions:

1. Combine sweet potatoes, parsnips, turnips, leeks, smoked paprika, and rosemary in the slow cooker
2. Heat olive oil in a pan and sauté leeks until golden, then add to the cooker
3. Pour vegetable broth, diced tomatoes, and apple cider vinegar over the vegetables
4. Season with salt and pepper
5. Cover and cook on low for 6 hr

Tips:

- Stir well before serving to mix the flavors
- Can be garnished with fresh parsley or a dollop of yogurt for a creamier texture
- Excellent served over cooked quinoa for added protein

Nutritional Values: Calories: 210, Fat: 3g, Carbs: 45g, Protein: 5g, Sugar: 15g, Sodium: 690 mg, Potassium: 1060 mg, Cholesterol: 0 mg

Chickpea Tagine with Apricots and Almonds

Preparation Time: 25 min
Cooking Time: 4 hr
Mode of Cooking: Slow Cooking
Servings: 4
Ingredients:

- 1 lb. dried chickpeas, soaked overnight and drained
- 3 cups water
- 1 onion, chopped
- 2 cloves garlic, minced
- 1 Tbsp ginger, freshly grated
- 1 cinnamon stick
- 4 cardamon pods
- 1 tsp cumin seeds
- 1 Tbsp coriander powder
- 1 cup dried apricots, chopped
- ½ cup almonds, toasted and slivered
- 2 Tbsp honey
- 2 Tbsp olive oil

Directions:

1. In a skillet, toast cumin seeds, cardamon pods until fragrant
2. Heat olive oil in the same skillet and sauté onions, garlic, and ginger until soft
3. Transfer mixture to a slow cooker along with soaked chickpeas, cinnamon stick, coriander powder, apricots, almonds, and water
4. Drizzle honey over the top
5. Cook on low for 4 hr

Tips:

- Stir the tagine before serving and remove the cinnamon stick
- Serve with couscous or flatbread for a complete meal
- Garnish with fresh cilantro for an added burst of flavor

Nutritional Values: Calories: 380, Fat: 10g, Carbs: 65g, Protein: 12g, Sugar: 20g, Sodium: 30 mg, Potassium: 900 mg, Cholesterol: 0 mg

SLOW-COOKED MEDITERRANEAN CHICKEN

Preparation Time: 10 min
Cooking Time: 7 hr
Mode of Cooking: Slow Cooking
Servings: 6
Ingredients:

- 6 boneless chicken breasts
- 1 cup kalamata olives, pitted
- 1 cup cherry tomatoes
- 1/2 cup artichoke hearts, quartered
- 3 cloves garlic, minced
- 1 lemon, juiced and zest
- 1 Tbsp dried oregano
- 2 Tbsp olive oil
- Salt and pepper to taste
- 1/2 cup white wine

Directions:

1. Place chicken breasts in the slow cooker
2. Top with kalamata olives, cherry tomatoes, artichoke hearts, and minced garlic
3. Sprinkle with lemon zest, juice, dried oregano, salt, and pepper
4. Drizzle olive oil and white wine over the top
5. Cover and cook on low for 7 hr

Tips:

- Serve this dish with a side of cooked orzo or rice for a hearty meal
- Drizzle some of the cooking juices over the chicken when serving to enhance flavors
- Garnish with fresh basil or parsley for a fresh touch

Nutritional Values: Calories: 220, Fat: 8g, Carbs: 6g, Protein: 28g, Sugar: 2g, Sodium: 590 mg, Potassium: 340 mg, Cholesterol: 75 mg

HERB-INFUSED BEEF POT ROAST

Preparation Time: 20 min.
Cooking Time: 8 hr.
Mode of Cooking: Slow Cooking
Servings: 6
Ingredients:

- 3 lb. chuck beef roast
- 1 large onion, sliced
- 4 cloves garlic, minced
- 2 carrots, chopped
- 2 celery stalks, chopped
- 3 cups beef broth
- 1 tsp dried thyme
- 1 tsp dried rosemary
- 2 bay leaves
- Salt and pepper to taste

Directions:

1. Season beef with salt and pepper and place in slow cooker
2. Top with onion, garlic, carrots, and celery
3. Add thyme, rosemary, and bay leaves
4. Pour beef broth over ingredients
5. Cook on low for 8 hr. or until beef is tender and falls apart easily

Tips:

- Use fresh herbs for a more intense flavor if available
- Remove bay leaves before serving
- Shred beef in the pot to soak up the flavors

Nutritional Values: Calories: 510, Fat: 34g, Carbs: 15g, Protein: 40g, Sugar: 5g, Sodium: 390 mg, Potassium: 850 mg, Cholesterol: 120 mg

Chapter 6: Snacks and Sides

Navigating the journey of managing diverticulitis, we encounter many moments where a soothing snack or a well-crafted side dish makes all the difference. This chapter is devoted to these smaller, yet significant, culinary delights that not only comply with your dietary needs but also bring joy and flavor to your everyday meals.

Imagine settling down for a mid-afternoon break where instead of reaching for something you know you shouldn't eat, you choose a snack that actively soothes your gut. Or picture a family dinner where the side dishes are met with smiles, not sighs, because they're both delicious and designed to ease digestion. That's what we aim to offer you here: a range of snacks and sides that you can enjoy without hesitation, focusing on ingredients that are gentle on the gut and inviting to the palate.

It's crucial to find joy in the food we can eat, not just mourn what we cannot. This chapter introduces choices like healing teas that double as delightful warm drinks, side dishes rich in soothing fibers without causing discomfort, and snacks that pack both nutrition and flavor, carefully avoiding those ingredients known to trigger flare-ups. Each recipe is crafted to ensure that it's not just safe but also a pleasure to eat.

The focus here is on balance—balancing fiber, respecting the limits of FODMAPs, and incorporating anti-inflammatory foods. We explore how simple ingredients like ginger, peppermint, and turmeric can transform a basic snack into a healing remedy. There's power in pairing the right flavors and foods, and this section of the book is dedicated to teaching you that art.

Through these pages, you'll discover that managing your diet for diverticulitis doesn't mean sacrificing the joy of eating. It means adapting and transforming your approach to snacks and sides, turning necessary restrictions into an opportunity for culinary creativity and gut health rejuvenation.

6.1 Gentle and Nutritious Snacks

Yogurt and Fruit Parfait

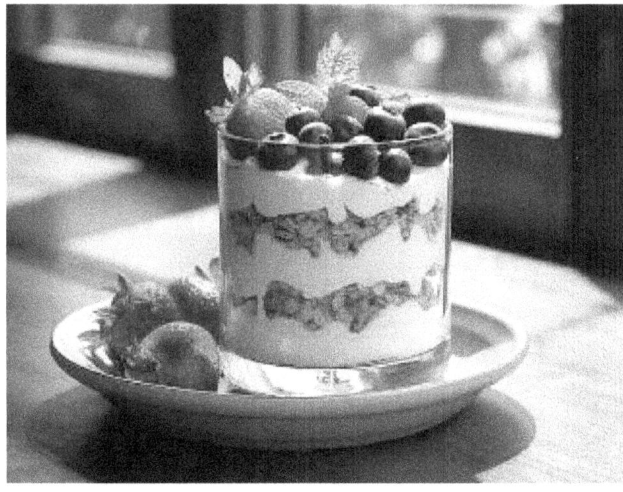

Preparation Time: 10 min
Cooking Time: none
Mode of Cooking: No Cooking
Servings: 2
Ingredients:

- 1 cup Greek yogurt, plain
- ½ cup granola, gluten-free
- ¼ cup blueberries, fresh
- ¼ cup strawberries, sliced
- 1 Tbsp honey, raw

Directions:

1. Layer half the Greek yogurt in two glasses
2. Add a layer of granola followed by a layer of blueberries and strawberries
3. Repeat the layering with the remaining yogurt and top with honey

Tips:

- Serve immediately for best flavor and texture
- Personalize with your favorite fruits or a sprinkle of cinnamon for added spice

Nutritional Values: Calories: 210, Fat: 2g, Carbs: 44g, Protein: 12g, Sugar: 30g, Sodium: 70 mg, Potassium: 300 mg, Cholesterol: 10 mg

Classic Hummus and Veggie Sticks

Preparation Time: 15 min
Cooking Time: none
Mode of Cooking: No Cooking
Servings: 4
Ingredients:

- 1 can chickpeas, drained and rinsed
- 2 Tbsp tahini, well stirred
- 1 garlic clove, minced
- 2 Tbsp lemon juice, fresh
- 3 Tbsp extra virgin olive oil
- ½ tsp cumin, ground
- Salt to taste
- Assorted veggie sticks (carrot, celery, bell pepper)

Directions:

1. Combine chickpeas, tahini, garlic, lemon juice, olive oil, cumin, and salt in a food processor
2. Blend until smooth and creamy
3. Adjust seasoning if necessary and transfer to a serving bowl

Tips:

- Opt for organic vegetables to dip
- Add a pinch of paprika on top of the hummus before serving for a touch of spice
- Refrigerate hummus for 1 hr before serving to enhance flavors

Nutritional Values: Calories: 170, Fat: 9g, Carbs: 20g, Protein: 5g, Sugar: 3g, Sodium: 400 mg, Potassium: 240 mg, Cholesterol: 0 mg

Rice Cakes with Almond Butter and Banana

Preparation Time: 5 min
Cooking Time: none
Mode of Cooking: No Cooking
Servings: 2
Ingredients:

- 2 rice cakes, whole grain
- 2 Tbsp almond butter, smooth
- 1 banana, thinly sliced
- 1 tsp chia seeds

Directions:

1. Spread almond butter evenly on each rice cake
2. Layer sliced banana on top of almond butter
3. Sprinkle chia seeds over the banana slices

Tips:

- Store leftover almond butter in a cool, dry place for optimal freshness
- Slice bananas just before serving to prevent browning
- Opt for freshly ground almond butter for best taste

Nutritional Values: Calories: 210, Fat: 9g, Carbs: 29g, Protein: 4g, Sugar: 10g, Sodium: 55 mg, Potassium: 450 mg, Cholesterol: 0 mg

Cucumber Rolls with Herbed Cream Cheese

Preparation Time: 20 min
Cooking Time: none
Mode of Cooking: No Cooking
Servings: 6
Ingredients:

- 1 large cucumber, peeled and thinly sliced lengthwise
- 4 oz cream cheese, softened
- 1 Tbsp dill, fresh, chopped
- 1 Tbsp chives, fresh, chopped
- Salt and pepper to taste
- ¼ red bell pepper, finely diced

Directions:

1. Combine cream cheese, dill, chives, salt, and pepper in a bowl
2. Mix until well combined
3. Lay cucumber slices on a flat surface

4. Spread a thin layer of the herbed cream cheese on each slice
5. Place a few pieces of red bell pepper at one end of each cucumber slice
6. Roll up tightly

Tips:

- Serve immediately or chill before serving for a firmer bite
- Use a vegetable peeler for even and thin cucumber slices
- If cream cheese mixture is too thick, soften with a teaspoon of milk

Nutritional Values: Calories: 70, Fat: 5g, Carbs: 4g, Protein: 1g, Sugar: 2g, Sodium: 80 mg, Potassium: 150 mg, Cholesterol: 15 mg

Yogurt and Spiced Pear Parfait

Preparation Time: 15 min
Cooking Time: none
Mode of Cooking: No Cooking
Servings: 2
Ingredients:

- 1 C. Greek yogurt, plain
- 1 pear, ripe, cubed
- 1/4 C. walnuts, toasted and chopped
- 1/2 tsp ground cinnamon
- 1 Tbsp honey
- 2 Tbsp old-fashioned oats, dry-toasted

Directions:

1. Mix Greek yogurt with honey and cinnamon in a bowl
2. Layer half of the yogurt mixture into two glasses
3. Add a layer of cubed pears to each glass
4. Sprinkle toasted oats and walnuts
5. Repeat the layering process finishing with a sprinkle of cinnamon on top

Tips:

- Serve immediately for best texture or store in refrigerator to allow flavors to meld
- Use pears that are just ripe for natural sweetness and gentle texture

Nutritional Values: Calories: 220, Fat: 8g, Carbs: 30g, Protein: 12g, Sugar: 20g, Sodium: 60 mg, Potassium: 170 mg, Cholesterol: 10 mg

6.2 Healing Side Dishes

Steamed Carrot Ribbons with Lemon and Dill

Preparation Time: Prep Time: 15 min.
Cooking Time: 5 min.
Mode of Cooking: Steaming
Servings: 4
Ingredients:

- 6 large carrots, peeled and sliced into thin ribbons
- 2 Tbsp fresh dill, chopped
- Zest of 1 lemon
- 1 Tbsp lemon juice
- 2 Tbsp extra virgin olive oil
- Salt and pepper to taste

Directions:

1. Peel and slice carrots into thin ribbons using a vegetable peeler
2. Steam carrot ribbons for about 5 minutes until tender but still crisp
3. In a mixing bowl, combine steamed carrots with fresh dill, lemon zest, lemon juice, and extra virgin olive oil
4. Season with salt and pepper to taste
5. Toss gently to combine all ingredients evenly

Tips:

- Add a splash of orange juice for a sweet citrus twist
- Garnish with additional fresh herbs such as parsley or chives for enhanced flavor and presentation

Nutritional Values: Calories: 90, Fat: 7g, Carbs: 7g, Protein: 1g, Sugar: 3g, Sodium: 70 mg, Potassium: 210 mg, Cholesterol: 0 mg

Mashed Sweet Potatoes with Cilantro and Lime

Preparation Time: Prep Time: 10 min.
Cooking Time: 20 min.
Mode of Cooking: Boiling
Servings: 4
Ingredients:

- 4 medium sweet potatoes, peeled and cubed
- 2 Tbsp unsalted butter
- 1/4 cup light cream
- Juice and zest of 1 lime
- 1/4 cup cilantro, finely chopped
- Salt and black pepper to taste

Directions:

1. Boil sweet potatoes in salted water until tender, about 20 minutes
2. Drain and return potatoes to the pot
3. Add unsalted butter and light cream, then mash until smooth
4. Stir in lime juice, lime zest, and chopped cilantro
5. Season with salt and black pepper to taste
6. Mix well until all ingredients are fully incorporated

Tips:

- Serve with a dollop of Greek yogurt on top for extra cream, and for vibrant taste and health benefits

Nutritional Values: Calories: 200, Fat: 7g, Carbs: 33g, Protein: 2g, Sugar: 7g, Sodium: 85 mg, Potassium: 475 mg, Cholesterol: 20 mg

Roasted Zucchini with Parmesan and Herbs

Preparation Time: Prep Time: 10 min.
Cooking Time: 15 min.
Mode of Cooking: Roasting
Servings: 4
Ingredients:

- 4 medium zucchini, sliced into 1/4 inch thick rounds
- 1/4 cup grated Parmesan cheese
- 1 Tbsp olive oil
- 1 tsp dried basil
- 1 tsp dried oregano
- 1/2 tsp garlic powder
- Salt and pepper to taste

Directions:

1. Preheat oven to 450°F (230°C)
2. Toss zucchini rounds with olive oil, basil, oregano, garlic powder, salt, and pepper
3. Spread in a single layer on a baking sheet
4. Sprinkle grated Parmesan cheese over the top
5. Roast in the preheated oven for about 15 minutes, or until golden and tender

Tips:

- Garnish with fresh basil leaves before serving
- Rotate the baking sheet halfway through cooking for even roasting

Nutritional Values: Calories: 100, Fat: 6g, Carbs: 8g, Protein: 4g, Sugar: 5g, Sodium: 160 mg, Potassium: 510 mg, Cholesterol: 5 mg

Ginger-Turmeric Steamed Carrots

Preparation Time: 10 min
Cooking Time: 15 min
Mode of Cooking: Steaming
Servings: 4
Ingredients:

- 6 medium carrots, peeled and sliced
- 1 Tbsp fresh ginger, grated
- 1 tsp turmeric powder
- 1 Tbsp olive oil
- Salt and pepper to taste
- Fresh parsley, chopped for garnish

Directions:

1. Fill steamer with water and bring to a boil
2. Mix carrots with ginger, turmeric, olive oil, salt, and pepper in a steaming basket
3. Place basket in steamer, cover, and steam for 15 min. or until carrots are tender
4. Garnish with fresh parsley before serving

Tips:

- Serve immediately for best flavor and texture
- Adding a squeeze of fresh lemon juice enhances the antioxidants absorption
- Ideal pairing with grilled fish or poultry

Nutritional Values: Calories: 90, Fat: 4.5g, Carbs: 12g, Protein: 1g, Sugar: 5g, Sodium: 70mg, Potassium: 360mg, Cholesterol: 0mg

Cinnamon Maple Mashed Sweet Potatoes

Preparation Time: 20 min
Cooking Time: 35 min
Mode of Cooking: Boiling and Mashing
Servings: 4
Ingredients:

- 4 large sweet potatoes, peeled and cubed
- 2 Tbsp unsalted butter
- 1/4 cup maple syrup
- 1/2 tsp ground cinnamon
- 1/4 cup milk
- Salt to taste

Directions:

1. Place sweet potatoes in a large pot of salted water
2. Bring to a boil and cook until tender, about 25 min.
3. Drain well and return to pot
4. Add butter, maple syrup, cinnamon, and milk to the pot
5. Mash until smooth and well combined
6. Season with salt

Tips:

- Can be made ahead and reheated, which enhances the flavors
- A pinch of nutmeg can add a warm, spicy note
- Substitute almond milk for a dairy-free version

Nutritional Values: Calories: 295, Fat: 6g, Carbs: 58g, Protein: 3g, Sugar: 15g, Sodium: 85mg, Potassium: 780mg, Cholesterol: 15mg

6.3 Digestive Teas and Drinks

Gentle Ginger Tea

Preparation Time: 5 min
Cooking Time: 10 min
Mode of Cooking: Simmering
Servings: 2
Ingredients:

- 2 cups water
- 1 Tbsp fresh ginger, peeled and thinly sliced
- 1 tsp honey
- 1 Tbsp lemon juice
- A pinch of ground cinnamon

Directions:

1. Bring water to a boil
2. Add ginger slices and simmer for 10 min
3. Remove from heat and strain into cups
4. Stir in honey, lemon juice, and cinnamon

Tips:

- Enjoy this tea warm for the best soothing effect
- Add a slice of lemon for an extra zing and vitamin C boost

Nutritional Values: Calories: 25, Fat: 0g, Carbs: 6g, Protein: 0g, Sugar: 5g, Sodium: 1 mg, Potassium: 10 mg, Cholesterol: 0 mg

Chamomile-Lemon Balm Tea

Preparation Time: 5 min
Cooking Time: 10 min
Mode of Cooking: Steeping
Servings: 2
Ingredients:

- 1 Tbsp chamomile flowers
- 1 Tbsp lemon balm leaves
- 2 cups boiling water
- 1 tsp honey (optional)

Directions:

1. Pour boiling water over chamomile flowers and lemon balm leaves in a teapot
2. Cover and let steep for 10 min
3. Strain tea into cups and sweeten with honey if desired

Tips:

- Serve this tea before bedtime to aid in relaxation and digestion
- Can be enjoyed cold for a refreshing daytime drink

Nutritional Values: Calories: 2, Fat: 0g, Carbs: 0.5g, Protein: 0g, Sugar: 0g (1g if honey is added), Sodium: 0 mg, Potassium: 9 mg, Cholesterol: 0 mg

Refreshing Cucumber Water

Preparation Time: 5 min
Cooking Time: none
Mode of Cooking: Infusion
Servings: 4
Ingredients:

- 1 medium cucumber, thinly sliced
- 8 cups water
- 2 Tbsp mint leaves, roughly torn
- 1 Tbsp lime juice

Directions:

1. Combine all ingredients in a large pitcher
2. Stir gently to mix flavors
3. Chill in the refrigerator for at least 1 hr to allow the cucumber and mint flavors to infuse the water

Tips:

- Add ice cubes before serving for extra refreshment
- Garnish with lime slices or additional mint leaves for a more decorative presentation

Nutritional Values: Calories: 0, Fat: 0g, Carbs: 0g, Protein: 0g, Sugar: 0g, Sodium: 0 mg, Potassium: 76 mg, Cholesterol: 0 mg

Soothing Licorice Root Tea

Preparation Time: 5 min
Cooking Time: 15 min
Mode of Cooking: Simmering
Servings: 2
Ingredients:

- 1 Tbsp licorice root, chopped
- 2 cups water
- 1 cinnamon stick
- 1 cardamom pod, cracked open
- 1 clove

Directions:

1. Combine licorice root, cinnamon stick, cardamom pod, and clove with water in a small saucepan
2. Bring to a boil, then reduce heat and simmer for 15 min
3. Strain the tea into cups

Tips:

- Drink warm to maximize the soothing effects on the throat and digestive system
- Add a splash of almond milk for a creamier texture and flavor

Nutritional Values: Calories: 5, Fat: 0g, Carbs: 1g, Protein: 0g, Sugar: 0g, Sodium: 0 mg, Potassium: 35 mg, Cholesterol: 0 mg

Ginger Root Tea

Preparation Time: 10 min.
Cooking Time: 20 min.
Mode of Cooking: Simmering
Servings: 4
Ingredients:

- 2 inches fresh ginger root, thinly sliced
- 4 cups water
- 1 Tbsp honey
- 1 lemon, juiced

Directions:

1. Bring water to a boil in a saucepan
2. Add ginger slices and reduce heat to a simmer for 20 minutes
3. Remove from heat and stir in lemon juice and honey
4. Strain into cups and serve warm

Tips:

- Add a cinnamon stick during simmering for a spicy twist
- Use fresh orange juice instead of lemon for a different flavor
- Honey can be substituted with maple syrup for a vegan option

Nutritional Values: Calories: 40, Fat: 0g, Carbs: 10g, Protein: 0g, Sugar: 9g, Sodium: 5 mg, Potassium: 49 mg, Cholesterol: 0 mg

Chapter 7: Baking for Better Digestion

The aroma of freshly baked bread, the crackle of a warm cookie fresh out of the oven—these are comforts many fear they must sacrifice when navigating the strictures of a diverticulitis-friendly diet. Yet, in this chapter, I'm delighted to share that such delights are not only possible but can even be beneficial to your gut health if prepared thoughtfully.

Baking for better digestion is an art and science that harnesses the soothing magic of the oven to produce eats that both heal and hearten. It's about transforming the kitchen from a place of dietary restrictions into a sanctuary where healing and enjoyment coalesce. Here, each recipe is crafted to minimize distress to your digestive system while maximizing nutritional benefits, particularly focusing on enhancing digestive health with ingredients that are not only safe but supportive in managing diverticulitis.

Imagine indulging in a slice of fiber-rich banana bread that not only satiates your sweet tooth but also nurtures your gut flora. Or picture yourself biting into a savory, golden biscuit that pairs perfectly with a hearty, homemade soup without causing any discomfort. These are not mere daydreams but achievable, everyday treats designed to support your digestive system's needs.

The secret to successful baking in a diverticulitis diet lies in the careful selection of ingredients that keep inflammation at bay while providing ample flavor and texture. For instance, whole grains and seeds that are normally avoided during flare-ups can be reintroduced gradually in baked goods as part of a long-term maintenance phase, prepared in ways that make them more digestible.

Moreover, this chapter does more than just offer recipes; it's a source of empowerment. Here, you'll learn to create dishes that replace feelings of limitation with liberation—each recipe is a step towards reclaiming the joy of baking and the comfort of traditional home-cooked delights, reimagined for your health. Whether you're a novice baker or a seasoned pro, these recipes are designed to be straightforward, satisfying, and safe, ensuring that your journey towards digestive health is as enjoyable as it is healing.

7.1 Fiber-Friendly Breads

Flaxseed and Chia Whole Wheat Bread

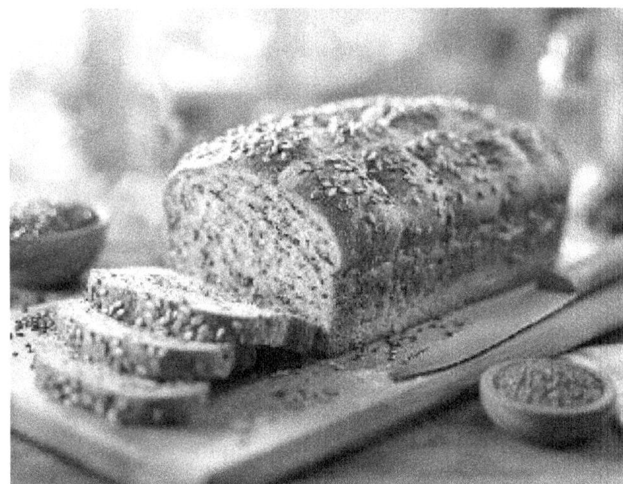

Preparation Time: 15 min
Cooking Time: 35 min
Mode of Cooking: Baking
Servings: 1 loaf

Ingredients:

- 2 cups whole wheat flour
- 1 tbsp sugar
- 1 packet dry yeast
- ¾ cup warm water
- ¼ cup ground flaxseed
- 2 tbsp chia seeds
- 1 tsp salt
- 1 tbsp olive oil

Directions:

1. Mix sugar, warm water, and yeast in a bowl and let sit until frothy
2. In a separate bowl, combine whole wheat flour, flaxseed, chia seeds, and salt

3. Add the yeast mixture and olive oil to the dry ingredients and knead until smooth
4. Let the dough rise in a warm place for 1 hr
5. Punch down the dough and shape into a loaf
6. Place in a greased loaf pan and let rise for another 30 min
7. Preheat oven to 375°F (190°C)
8. Bake the bread for 35 min

Tips:

- Use honey instead of sugar for a natural sweetness
- Brush the top with milk before baking for a golden crust

Nutritional Values: Calories: 120, Fat: 3g, Carbs: 20g, Protein: 4g, Sugar: 1g, Sodium: 200 mg, Potassium: 89 mg, Cholesterol: 0 mg

Gluten-Free Chia Banana Bread

Preparation Time: 20 min
Cooking Time: 45 min
Mode of Cooking: Baking
Servings: 1 loaf
Ingredients:

- 2 cups gluten-free oat flour
- 1 tsp baking powder
- ½ tsp baking soda
- ¼ tsp salt
- 1 cup ripe bananas, mashed
- 3 Tbsp honey
- ¾ cup almond milk
- 4 Tbsp coconut oil, melted
- 2 tsp vanilla extract
- ½ cup chia seeds

Directions:

1. In a large bowl, mix oat flour, baking powder, baking soda, and salt
2. In another bowl, whisk together mashed bananas, honey, almond milk, melted coconut oil, and vanilla extract
3. Combine wet and dry ingredients and stir until just mixed
4. Fold in chia seeds
5. Pour batter into a greased loaf pan
6. Preheat oven to 350°F (175°C)
7. Bake for 45 min

Tips:

- Allow the bread to cool in the pan for 10 min before transferring to a wire rack to cool completely
- Adding a pinch of cinnamon can enhance flavor

Nutritional Values: Calories: 160, Fat: 6g, Carbs: 24g, Protein: 3g, Sugar: 8g, Sodium: 230 mg, Potassium: 75 mg, Cholesterol: 0 mg

Oat Bran and Apple Cinnamon Muffins

Preparation Time: 15 min
Cooking Time: 20 min
Mode of Cooking: Baking
Servings: 12 muffins
Ingredients:

- 2 cups oat bran
- 1 tbsp ground cinnamon
- ½ tsp salt
- 1 tbsp baking powder
- 1 cup unsweetened applesauce
- 2 eggs, beaten
- ¼ cup maple syrup
- ½ cup milk
- 1/4 cup olive oil
- 1 tsp vanilla extract
- 1 cup diced apples

Directions:

1. Combine oat bran, cinnamon, salt, and baking powder in a bowl
2. In another bowl, mix applesauce, beaten eggs, maple syrup, milk, olive oil, and vanilla extract

3. Add wet ingredients to dry ingredients and stir until just combined
4. Fold in diced apples
5. Spoon batter into greased muffin tins
6. Preheat oven to 400°F (204°C)
7. Bake for 20 min

Tips:

- Try using pear instead of apple for a different flavor profile
- Sprinkle the top with rolled oats before baking for added texture

Nutritional Values: Calories: 140, Fat: 5g, Carbs: 22g, Protein: 4g, Sugar: 6g, Sodium: 150 mg, Potassium: 103 mg, Cholesterol: 31 mg

SORGHUM FLOUR CARROT BREAD

Preparation Time: 20 min
Cooking Time: 50 min
Mode of Cooking: Baking
Servings: 1 loaf
Ingredients:

- 2 cups sorghum flour
- 1 tsp baking powder
- ½ tsp baking soda
- ¼ tsp salt
- 1 tsp cinnamon
- ½ cup sugar
- 1 cup grated carrots
- ¾ cup buttermilk
- ½ cup vegetable oil
- 2 eggs
- 1 tsp vanilla extract

Directions:

1. Mix sorghum flour, baking powder, baking soda, salt, cinnamon, and sugar in a large bowl
2. In another bowl, combine grated carrots, buttermilk, vegetable oil, eggs, and vanilla extract
3. Add wet ingredients to dry ingredients and mix until well blended
4. Pour batter into a greased loaf pan
5. Preheat oven to 350°F (175°C)
6. Bake for 50 min

Tips:

- Add a handful of walnuts or pecans for extra crunch and flavor
- Sprinkle the top with raw sugar before baking for a crispy crust

Nutritional Values: Calories: 180, Fat: 8g, Carbs: 26g, Protein: 3g, Sugar: 12g, Sodium: 220 mg, Potassium: 77 mg, Cholesterol: 53 mg

WHOLE WHEAT CHIA SEED LOAF

Preparation Time: 15 min
Cooking Time: 35 min
Mode of Cooking: Baking
Servings: 1 loaf
Ingredients:

- 3 cups whole wheat flour
- 1 Tbsp instant yeast
- 1 Tbsp honey
- 1½ cups warm water
- 2 Tbsp olive oil
- 1 tsp salt
- ¼ cup chia seeds

Directions:

1. Combine honey, warm water, and yeast in a large bowl and let sit until foamy about 5 min
2. Mix in olive oil, salt, and whole wheat flour gradually until dough begins to form
3. Knead the dough on a lightly floured surface for about 10 min
4. Roll dough into a ball and return to bowl, cover with a damp cloth and let it rise in a warm place for 1 hr until doubled in size
5. Punch down the dough and knead in chia seeds

6. Shape the dough into a loaf and place into a greased loaf pan
7. Cover and let rise for another 30 min
8. Preheat oven to 375°F (190°C)
9. Bake for 35 min until the crust is golden and loaf sounds hollow when tapped

Tips:

- Oil your hands when kneading in the chia seeds to prevent sticking
- Slice with a serrated knife for cleaner cuts

Nutritional Values: Calories: 180, Fat: 4g, Carbs: 30g, Protein: 6g, Sugar: 2g, Sodium: 200 mg, Potassium: 100 mg, Cholesterol: 0 mg

7.2 Digestive-Boosting Cookies and Bars

Ginger-Flaxseed Oatmeal Bars

Preparation Time: 15 min
Cooking Time: 25 min
Mode of Cooking: Baking
Servings: 16
Ingredients:

- 2 cups rolled oats
- 1 cup flaxseed meal
- 1/2 cup almond milk
- 1/3 cup maple syrup
- 1/4 cup crystallized ginger, finely chopped
- 1/4 cup unsweetened apple sauce
- 1 tsp vanilla extract
- 1/2 tsp ground cinnamon
- 1/4 tsp salt

Directions:

1. Preheat oven to 350°F (175°C)
2. Mix oats and flaxseed meal in a large bowl
3. In a separate bowl, blend almond milk, maple syrup, apple sauce, and vanilla extract
4. Combine wet and dry ingredients, add crystallized ginger, cinnamon, and salt, mix well
5. Spread the mixture evenly in a parchment-lined baking pan
6. Bake until the edges are golden brown and the center is set

Tips:

- Cut into bars when cooled for a cleaner slice
- Store in an airtight container at room temperature to maintain freshness

Nutritional Values: Calories: 120, Fat: 4g, Carbs: 18g, Protein: 3g, Sugar: 7g, Sodium: 40 mg, Potassium: 105 mg, Cholesterol: 0 mg

Chewy Banana Nut Quinoa Bars

Preparation Time: 20 min
Cooking Time: 30 min
Mode of Cooking: Baking
Servings: 12
Ingredients:

- 1 cup quinoa flakes
- 1 cup ripe bananas, mashed
- 1/2 cup walnuts, chopped
- 1/4 cup honey
- 1/4 cup coconut oil, melted
- 2 Tbsp chia seeds
- 1 tsp cinnamon
- 1/2 tsp nutmeg
- 1/4 tsp salt

Directions:

1. Preheat oven to 375°F (190°C)
2. Mix quinoa flakes, chia seeds, cinnamon, nutmeg, and salt in a bowl
3. In another bowl, combine mashed bananas, honey, and melted coconut oil Stir wet ingredients into dry ingredients, then fold in chopped walnuts
4. Pour into a lined baking tray and smooth the top
5. Bake until the edges start to brown and a toothpick comes out clean from the center

Tips:

- Slice while warm for easier cutting
- These bars can be frozen for up to a month for long-term enjoyment

Nutritional Values: Calories: 180, Fat: 8g, Carbs: 24g, Protein: 4g, Sugar: 10g, Sodium: 55 mg, Potassium: 134 mg, Cholesterol: 0 mg

Almond-Coconut Flour Cookies

Preparation Time: 10 min
Cooking Time: 12 min
Mode of Cooking: Baking
Servings: 18
Ingredients:

- 1 1/2 cups almond flour
- 1/2 cup coconut flour
- 1/3 cup coconut oil, melted
- 1/4 cup honey
- 2 tsp almond extract
- 1/2 tsp baking soda
- 1/4 tsp salt

Directions:

1. Preheat oven to 350°F (175°C)
2. Whisk together almond flour, coconut flour, baking soda, and salt in a bowl
3. Stir in melted coconut oil, honey, and almond extract until dough forms
4. Scoop dough by tablespoon onto a baking sheet lined with parchment paper
5. Flatten each cookie slightly
6. Bake until edges are golden brown

Tips:

- Allow cookies to cool on the baking sheet for 10 minutes to set properly
- Store in an airtight container to keep them moist
- Adapt sweetness by adding or reducing honey according to taste

Nutritional Values: Calories: 130, Fat: 9g, Carbs: 11g, Protein: 3g, Sugar: 6g, Sodium: 55 mg, Potassium: 12 mg, Cholesterol: 0 mg

Pumpkin Seed and Cranberry Energy Bites

Preparation Time: 15 min
Cooking Time: none
Mode of Cooking: No Cooking
Servings: 20
Ingredients:

- 1 cup pumpkin seeds
- 1/2 cup dried cranberries, unsweetened
- 1/2 cup rolled oats
- 1/4 cup sunflower seeds
- 1/4 cup honey
- 1 Tbsp chia seeds
- 1 Tbsp coconut oil
- 1 tsp vanilla extract
- 1/4 tsp salt

Directions:

1. Combine all ingredients in a large bowl
2. Mix well until the mixture is sticky and combined
3. Roll the mixture into small balls
4. Place on a tray and refrigerate until firm

Tips:

- These bites can be stored in the refrigerator for up to a week for best freshness
- Customize by adding different nuts or seeds according to your taste preferences

Nutritional Values: Calories: 100, Fat: 5g, Carbs: 12g, Protein: 3g, Sugar: 8g, Sodium: 50 mg, Potassium: 95 mg, Cholesterol: 0 mg

Ginger Turmeric Almond Flour Cookies

Preparation Time: 15 min
Cooking Time: 10 min
Mode of Cooking: Baking
Servings: 24

Ingredients:

- 2 cups almond flour
- 1 tsp ground ginger
- ½ tsp ground turmeric
- ¼ tsp sea salt
- 1 tsp baking powder
- ½ cup pure maple syrup
- 1 large egg
- 2 Tbsp coconut oil, melted
- 1 tsp vanilla extract

Directions:

1. Preheat oven to 375°F (190°C)
2. In a large bowl combine almond flour, ground ginger, ground turmeric, sea salt, and baking powder
3. In another bowl, whisk together maple syrup, egg, melted coconut oil, and vanilla extract
4. Combine wet and dry ingredients until a dough forms
5. Drop by spoonfuls onto a parchment-lined baking sheet, flattening slightly
6. Bake for 10 min or until edges are just golden

Tips:

- Try adding a pinch of black pepper to enhance turmeric absorption
- Allow cookies to cool on the baking sheet for 5 min before transferring to a wire rack

Nutritional Values: Calories: 95, Fat: 6g, Carbs: 8g, Protein: 2g, Sugar: 5g, Sodium: 30 mg, Potassium: 10 mg, Cholesterol: 10 mg

7.3 Gentle and Sweet Treats

Spiced Applesauce Cake

Preparation Time: 20 min.
Cooking Time: 45 min.
Mode of Cooking: Baking
Servings: 8

Ingredients:

- 2 C. whole wheat flour
- 1 C. unsweetened applesauce
- ¾ C. erythritol
- ½ C. olive oil
- 2 tsp. cinnamon
- 1 tsp. baking soda
- ½ tsp. nutmeg
- ¼ tsp. salt
- 1 tsp. vanilla extract
- 2 eggs

Directions:

1. Preheat oven to 350°F (175°C)
2. In a large bowl, combine erythritol, olive oil, eggs, and vanilla extract and beat until creamy
3. In another bowl, whisk together flour, baking soda, cinnamon, nutmeg, and salt
4. Gradually add dry ingredients to the wet ingredients, alternating with applesauce, until just combined
5. Pour batter into a greased 9-inch square baking pan
6. Bake for 45 min. or until a toothpick inserted comes out clean

Tips:

- Allow cake to cool completely before slicing
- Serve with a dollop of Greek yogurt for extra creaminess

Nutritional Values: Calories: 210, Fat: 10g, Carbs: 28g, Protein: 4g, Sugar: 12g, Sodium: 320 mg, Potassium: 98 mg, Cholesterol: 53 mg

Yogurt and Berry Tart with Almond Crust

Preparation Time: 30 min.
Cooking Time: 15 min.
Mode of Cooking: Baking
Servings: 8

Ingredients:

- 1½ C. almond flour
- ¼ C. coconut oil, melted
- 2 Tbsp. honey
- 1 tsp. almond extract
- 1½ C. Greek yogurt, plain
- 2 Tbsp. honey
- 1 tsp. vanilla extract
- 2 C. mixed berries (blueberries, raspberries, strawberries)

Directions:

1. Preheat oven to 375°F (190°C)
2. Mix almond flour, coconut oil, 2 Tbsp. honey, and almond extract to form the crust
3. Press mixture into a 9-inch tart pan and bake for 15 min.
4. Let cool completely
5. Combine Greek yogurt, 2 Tbsp. honey, and vanilla extract and spread over the cooled crust
6. Top with fresh berries and chill until set

Tips:

- Chill tart for at least 2 hours before serving for best consistency
- Opt for organic berries for enhanced flavor and nutrition

Nutritional Values: Calories: 250, Fat: 18g, Carbs: 18g, Protein: 7g, Sugar: 12g, Sodium: 20 mg, Potassium: 135 mg, Cholesterol: 10 mg

Steamed Cinnamon Pears

Preparation Time: 10 min.
Cooking Time: 20 min.
Mode of Cooking: Steaming
Servings: 4
Ingredients:

- 4 ripe pears, peeled and halved
- 1 C. water
- 2 Tbsp. honey
- 1 tsp. ground cinnamon
- ½ tsp. ground cloves

Directions:

1. Prepare steamer in a pot and bring water to a simmer
2. Mix honey, cinnamon, and cloves in a small bowl
3. Brush honey mixture over pear halves
4. Place pears in the steamer basket cut-side down
5. Cover and steam for 20 min. or until pears are tender

Tips:

- Serve warm with a sprinkle of crushed walnuts for added texture
- Accompany with a scoop of vanilla ice cream for a decadent treat

Nutritional Values: Calories: 120, Fat: 0.2g, Carbs: 31g, Protein: 0.5g, Sugar: 25g, Sodium: 5 mg, Potassium: 206 mg, Cholesterol: 0 mg

Applesauce Spice Cake

Preparation Time: 15 min.
Cooking Time: 35 min.
Mode of Cooking: Baking
Servings: 8
Ingredients:

- 2 C. all-purpose flour
- 1 tsp baking soda
- 1 tsp ground cinnamon
- 1/2 tsp ground nutmeg
- 1/4 tsp salt
- 1 C. unsweetened applesauce
- 1/3 C. vegetable oil
- 3/4 C. honey
- 2 large eggs
- 1 tsp vanilla extract
- 1/2 C. raisins
- 1/2 C. chopped walnuts

Directions:

1. Preheat oven to 350°F (175°C)
2. Grease a 9-inch square baking pan
3. In a large bowl, whisk together flour, baking soda, cinnamon, nutmeg, and salt
4. In another bowl, mix applesauce, oil, honey, eggs, and vanilla
5. Combine the wet and dry ingredients, then fold in raisins and walnuts
6. Pour into prepared pan and bake until a toothpick inserted in the center comes out clean

Tips:

- Keep cake covered to retain moisture
- Add a dollop of low-fat Greek yogurt on the side for extra richness

Nutritional Values: Calories: 270, Fat: 9g, Carbs: 46g, Protein: 4g, Sugar: 26g, Sodium: 210 mg, Potassium: 150 mg, Cholesterol: 40 mg

Yogurt and Berry Tart

Preparation Time: 20 min.
Cooking Time: none
Mode of Cooking: Refrigeration
Servings: 8
Ingredients:

- 2 C. graham cracker crumbs
- 1/3 C. melted unsalted butter
- 2 Tbsp sugar
- 2 C. low-fat Greek yogurt
- 1/4 C. honey
- 1 tsp vanilla extract
- 2 C. mixed fresh berries (strawberries, blueberries, raspberries)
- Mint leaves for garnish

Directions:

1. Mix graham cracker crumbs, butter, and sugar and press into the bottom of a tart pan to form a crust
2. Chill for 1 hr. to set
3. In a bowl, mix Greek yogurt, honey, and vanilla
4. Pour the yogurt mixture over the crust and smooth the surface
5. Arrange berries on top and garnish with mint leaves
6. Chill for at least 3 hrs. before serving

Tips:

- Use a mix of seasonal berries for best flavor and color contrast
- Store in refrigerator and serve chilled to maintain the firmness of the yogurt filling

Nutritional Values: Calories: 210, Fat: 8g, Carbs: 30g, Protein: 6g, Sugar: 18g, Sodium: 95 mg, Potassium: 170 mg, Cholesterol: 20 mg

Chapter 8: More Healing Soups and Broths

As we continue our journey towards a healthier, happier gut, we delve into the comforting world of soups and broths—a haven for those seeking solace and healing in the warmth of a bowl. Soups and broths, with their nurturing essence, have always been at the heart of dietary healing practices, and in the context of managing diverticulitis, they offer not just nourishment but gentle relief during times of recovery.

Imagine sitting down to a steaming bowl of broth, its steam carrying the wholesome aromas of bone marrow, tender vegetables, and fresh herbs. This isn't just food; it's medicine, crafted with the simplicity of ingredients known to soothe and repair. The process of preparing these broths and soups is almost as healing as consuming them, emphasizing a slow simmer that extracts every bit of goodness nature has to offer.

In this chapter, we explore a range of broths—including the robust, collagen-rich bone broths that provide the building blocks for a healthy gut lining, and the lighter vegetable souths that offer hydration and ease during times when your digestive system craves gentleness. We also venture into protein-rich soups that are designed to give you strength without overburdening a healing gut. Each recipe is developed with an eye towards balancing flavor with function; after all, soothing your digestive system should never mean sacrificing enjoyment of your meals.

Soups and broths also represent a practical solution to many of the challenges you face while managing diverticulitis. They can be made in large batches and stored, ensuring that a comforting meal is always at hand, even on your busiest days. They can be easily adjusted according to your dietary needs and tastes, making them a versatile option for the whole family.

As you explore these recipes, remember that each ingredient is chosen for its ability to support healing and offer relief. Whether it's the gelatin from bone broth sealing the gut, the anti-inflammatory properties of ginger, or the hydrating nature of cucumbers, know that you're nurturing your body with every spoonful. Step into your kitchen, and let's stir up both comfort and healing with these soul-satisfying soups and broths.

8.1 Bone Broths

Classic Beef Bone Broth

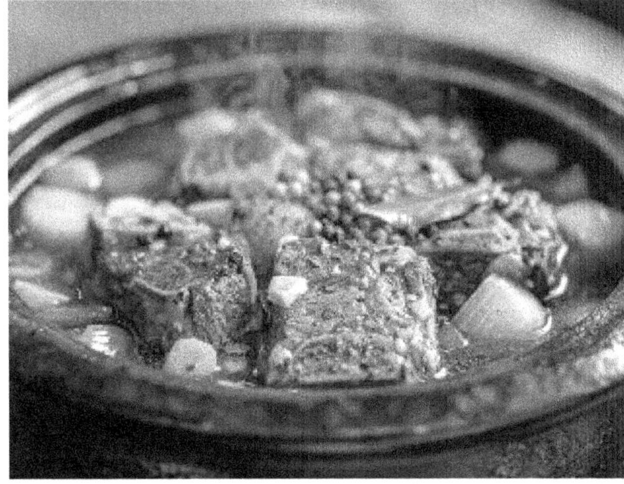

Preparation Time: 15 min
Cooking Time: 48 hr
Mode of Cooking: Slow Cooking
Servings: 8

Ingredients:

- 4 lb. beef bones with marrow
- 4 qt. water
- 2 carrots, chopped
- 1 onion, quartered
- 3 celery stalks, chopped
- 2 Tbsp apple cider vinegar
- 1 bay leaf
- 1 tsp black peppercorns
- 1 head garlic, halved horizontally

Directions:

1. Roast beef bones at 450°F (232°C) until golden, about 30 min
2. Place roasted bones and all other ingredients in a slow cooker

3. Cover with water
4. Cook on low heat for 48 hr
5. Strain the broth through a fine mesh sieve
6. Discard solids
7. Cool and skim off fat from the top of the broth

Tips:

- Chill the broth to help solidify the fat for easier removal
- Add a splash of vinegar to help extract minerals from the bones
- Freeze in small portions for easy use

Nutritional Values: Calories: 40, Fat: 0g, Carbs: 3g, Protein: 6g, Sugar: 1g, Sodium: 58 mg, Potassium: 210 mg, Cholesterol: 0 mg

Healing Chicken Bone Broth

Preparation Time: 10 min
Cooking Time: 24 hr
Mode of Cooking: Slow Cooking
Servings: 6
Ingredients:

- 3 lb. chicken bones
- 4 qt. water
- 2 carrots, chopped
- 2 onions, quartered
- 4 celery stalks, chopped
- 2 Tbsp apple cider vinegar
- 1 bunch parsley
- 1 bay leaf
- 1 tsp dried thyme
- 4 cloves garlic, crushed

Directions:

1. Roast chicken bones at 400°F (204°C) until browned, about 25 min
2. Place roasted bones and other ingredients except parsley in a slow cooker
3. Add water to cover
4. Cook on low for 24 hr
5. Add parsley in the last 30 min of cooking
6. Strain and discard solids
7. Skim fat from broth as needed

Tips:

- Store broth in glass jars to preserve freshness
- Use broth as a base for soups or sauces
- Incorporate fresh herbs towards the end of the cooking process to maintain their vibrant flavor and color

Nutritional Values: Calories: 30, Fat: 1g, Carbs: 2g, Protein: 4g, Sugar: 1g, Sodium: 70 mg, Potassium: 190 mg, Cholesterol: 10 mg

Vegan Mineral Broth

Preparation Time: 20 min
Cooking Time: 2 hr
Mode of Cooking: Simmering
Servings: 8
Ingredients:

- 4 qt. water
- 1 cup chopped leeks
- 2 cups chopped carrots
- 1 cup chopped celery
- 1 cup chopped potatoes
- 1 cup chopped parsley
- 2 Tbsp nutritional yeast
- 1 seaweed sheet
- 2 cups chopped kale
- 6 cloves garlic, minced
- 1 Tbsp turmeric
- 1 inch ginger, sliced

Directions:

1. Combine all ingredients in a large pot
2. Bring to a boil
3. Reduce to simmer for 2 hr
4. Strain the broth, pressing on the veggies to extract flavors
5. Discard solids

Tips:

- Add sea salt to taste after straining for better control of sodium content
- Store in the refrigerator and use within a week or freeze for up to 2 months
- Boost flavor with a dash of soy sauce or miso paste before serving

Nutritional Values: Calories: 70, Fat: 1g, Carbs: 16g, Protein: 3g, Sugar: 4g, Sodium: 100 mg, Potassium: 300 mg, Cholesterol: 0 mg

Nourishing Turkey Bone Broth

Preparation Time: 15 min
Cooking Time: 30 hr
Mode of Cooking: Slow Cooking
Servings: 8
Ingredients:

- 5 lb. turkey carcass, broken into small pieces
- 5 qt. water
- 3 carrots, chopped
- 2 onions, chopped
- 3 stalks celery, chopped
- 2 Tbsp apple cider vinegar
- 1 bay leaf
- 5 cloves garlic, smashed
- 1 tsp whole black peppercorns

Directions:

1. Roast turkey bones at 400°F (204°C) until well-browned, about 35 min
2. Place bones and all other ingredients in a large crock pot or slow cooker
3. Cover with water
4. Cook on low for 30 hr
5. Strain through a fine mesh strainer, discarding all solids
6. Skim off any excess fat from the surface

Tips:

- Reheat gently before serving to preserve nutrients
- Freeze in ice cube trays for small, easy-to-use portions
- Roasting the bones before simmering enhances the flavor and richness of the broth

Nutritional Values: Calories: 45, Fat: 1g, Carbs: 3g, Protein: 6g, Sugar: 1g, Sodium: 62 mg, Potassium: 250 mg, Cholesterol: 5 mg

Classic Beef Bone Broth

Preparation Time: 15 min
Cooking Time: 24 hr
Mode of Cooking: Simmering
Servings: 8
Ingredients:

- 4 lb. beef bones with marrow
- 4 qt. water
- 2 medium carrots, chopped
- 1 large onion, quartered
- 4 cloves garlic, smashed
- 2 Tbsp apple cider vinegar
- 1 tsp salt
- 1 tsp whole black peppercorns
- 3 bay leaves

Directions:

1. Place beef bones on a baking sheet and roast at 400°F (200°C) until golden, about 30 min
2. Transfer bones to a large pot and add water, ensuring bones are submerged
3. Add carrots, onion, garlic, apple cider vinegar, salt, peppercorns, and bay leaves
4. Bring to a boil, then reduce to a simmer and cover slightly ajar, cooking for 24 hr
5. Skim foam and excess fat occasionally
6. Strain the broth through a fine mesh sieve, discarding solids
7. Cool and store

Tips:

- Roast bones prior to simmering to enhance flavor

- Add vinegar to help extract minerals from the bones

Nutritional Values: Calories: 40, Fat: 0g, Carbs: 1g, Protein: 6g, Sugar: 0g, Sodium: 190 mg, Potassium: 0 mg, Cholesterol: 0 mg

8.2 Vegetable Soups

Carrot and Ginger Soup

Preparation Time: 15 min.
Cooking Time: 30 min.
Mode of Cooking: Stovetop
Servings: 4
Ingredients:

- 2 Tbsp olive oil
- 1 lb. carrots, peeled and chopped
- 2 Tbsp fresh ginger, minced
- 1 medium onion, chopped
- 4 cups vegetable broth
- 1 tsp salt
- 1/2 tsp black pepper
- 1 cup coconut milk

Directions:

1. Heat olive oil in a large pot over medium heat
2. Add onions and sauté until translucent
3. Stir in ginger and carrots and cook for another 5 min.
4. Pour in vegetable broth, bring to boil then simmer for 25 min. until carrots are tender
5. Puree the mixture using an immersion blender until smooth
6. Stir in coconut milk and heat through

Tips:

- Add a swirl of cream or a sprinkle of chopped parsley for garnish to enhance flavor and presentation
- Serve with a slice of whole-grain bread for a filling meal

Nutritional Values: Calories: 190, Fat: 11g, Carbs: 22g, Protein: 3g, Sugar: 10g, Sodium: 950 mg, Potassium: 690 mg, Cholesterol: 0 mg

Creamy Zucchini Soup

Preparation Time: 10 min.
Cooking Time: 25 min.
Mode of Cooking: Stovetop
Servings: 4
Ingredients:

- 1 Tbsp olive oil
- 1 white onion, diced
- 3 medium zucchini, chopped
- 1 potato, peeled and cubed
- 4 cups chicken broth
- Salt and pepper to taste
- 1/2 cup heavy cream
- Fresh basil leaves for garnish

Directions:

1. Heat olive oil in a pot over medium heat
2. Add onion and cook until soft
3. Incorporate zucchini and potato, cook for 5 min.
4. Add broth, season with salt and pepper, and simmer for 20 min.
5. Puree soup in batches in a blender until smooth, return to pot
6. Stir in heavy cream and heat through

Tips:

- Garnish with basil leaves before serving
- For a lighter version, substitute heavy cream with Greek yogurt
- Enjoy this soup either hot or chilled

Nutritional Values: Calories: 175, Fat: 12g, Carbs: 15g, Protein: 4g, Sugar: 5g, Sodium: 800 mg, Potassium: 470 mg, Cholesterol: 30 mg

Butternut Squash Soup

Preparation Time: 20 min.
Cooking Time: 40 min.
Mode of Cooking: Stovetop

Servings: 6

Ingredients:

- 2 Tbsp unsalted butter
- 1 medium onion, chopped
- 1 butternut squash, peeled, seeded, and cubed
- 1 apple, peeled and chopped
- 4 cups vegetable stock
- 1 tsp salt
- 1/2 tsp ground nutmeg
- 1/2 cup light cream
- Pumpkin seeds for garnish

Directions:

1. Melt butter in a large soup pot over medium heat
2. Add chopped onion and cook until translucent
3. Add squash and apple, cook for about 10 min.
4. Pour in vegetable stock, bring to a simmer and cook until squash is very soft, about 30 min.
5. Puree the mixture until smooth
6. Return to pot, stir in cream, season with nutmeg, and warm up

Tips:

- Top with toasted pumpkin seeds for added crunch and flavor
- This soup pairs well with a crusty piece of bread
- Add a bit of cinnamon for a deeper spice profile

Nutritional Values: Calories: 210, Fat: 9g, Carbs: 31g, Protein: 3g, Sugar: 12g, Sodium: 760 mg, Potassium: 790 mg, Cholesterol: 20 mg

Carrot and Ginger Zest Soup

Preparation Time: 15 min
Cooking Time: 30 min
Mode of Cooking: Simmering
Servings: 4

Ingredients:

- 1 lb. carrots, peeled and sliced
- 1 Tbsp extra virgin olive oil
- 1 onion, chopped
- 2 cloves garlic, minced
- 2 Tbsp fresh ginger, grated
- 4 cups vegetable broth
- 1 tsp lemon juice
- Salt and pepper to taste

Directions:

1. Heat olive oil in a large pot over medium heat
2. Saute onions, garlic, and ginger until onions are translucent
3. Add carrots and cook for 5 minutes
4. Pour in vegetable broth and bring to a boil
5. Reduce heat and simmer for 25 minutes or until carrots are tender
6. Puree the soup with an immersion blender until smooth
7. Stir in lemon juice, salt, and pepper

Tips:

- Serve with a dollop of yogurt for added creaminess
- Garnish with fresh parsley to enhance flavor

Nutritional Values: Calories: 120, Fat: 4g, Carbs: 20g, Protein: 2g, Sugar: 9g, Sodium: 720 mg, Potassium: 360 mg, Cholesterol: 0 mg

Creamy Zucchini Velvet Soup

Preparation Time: 10 min
Cooking Time: 20 min
Mode of Cooking: Simmering
Servings: 4

Ingredients:

- 3 medium zucchinis, chopped
- 1 Tbsp unsalted butter
- 1 small onion, diced
- 1 cup low-fat milk

- 1 cup vegetable stock
- Salt and white pepper to taste
- Nutmeg, a pinch

Directions:

1. Melt butter in a soup pot over medium heat
2. Add onions and saute until soft
3. Add chopped zucchinis and cook for 10 minutes
4. Pour in vegetable stock and milk, and season with salt, white pepper, and a pinch of nutmeg
5. Simmer for 10 minutes
6. Blend the mixture until creamy with an immersion blender

Tips:

- Add a sprinkle of grated Parmesan cheese for a richer flavor
- Serve hot, garnished with thin zucchini slices

Nutritional Values: Calories: 98, Fat: 5g, Carbs: 11g, Protein: 4g, Sugar: 7g, Sodium: 300 mg, Potassium: 510 mg, Cholesterol: 10 mg

8.3 Protein-Rich Soups

Chicken and Wild Rice Soup

Preparation Time: 15 min
Cooking Time: 35 min
Mode of Cooking: Stovetop
Servings: 4
Ingredients:

- 1 lb chicken breast, cubed
- 1 C. wild rice
- 1 large carrot, diced
- 1 celery stalk, diced
- 1 onion, chopped
- 2 cloves garlic, minced
- 4 C. low-sodium chicken broth
- 1 tsp dried thyme
- 1 tsp dried parsley
- ½ tsp black pepper
- 1 C. water
- 1 Tbsp olive oil

Directions:

1. Heat olive oil in a large pot over medium heat
2. Add onion, carrot, celery, and garlic, sauté until onions are translucent
3. Add cubed chicken breast and cook until browned
4. Stir in wild rice, chicken broth, water, thyme, parsley, and black pepper
5. Bring to a boil, then reduce heat and simmer for 25 min or until rice is tender

Tips:

- Stir occasionally to prevent sticking
- Can be served with a dollop of Greek yogurt for creaminess
- Add additional herbs for more flavor

Nutritional Values: Calories: 310, Fat: 6g, Carbs: 34g, Protein: 28g, Sugar: 3g, Sodium: 70 mg, Potassium: 410 mg, Cholesterol: 65 mg

Lentil and Spinach Soup

Preparation Time: 10 min
Cooking Time: 25 min
Mode of Cooking: Stovetop
Servings: 6
Ingredients:

- 1 C. dry green lentils
- 1 lb spinach, washed and chopped
- 1 large onion, chopped
- 2 carrots, diced
- 2 Tbsp tomato paste
- 1 tsp cumin
- 4 C. vegetable broth
- 2 C. water
- 2 Tbsp olive oil
- Salt and pepper to taste

Directions:

1. Heat olive oil in a soup pot over medium heat
2. Add onions and carrots, cook until softened
3. Stir in tomato paste and cumin, cook for 2 min
4. Add lentils, vegetable broth, and water, bring to a boil then simmer for 20 min
5. Add spinach, cook until wilted, season with salt and pepper

Tips:

- Serve hot, topped with a squeeze of lemon for added zest
- Perfect with a side of crusty bread
- Adjust seasoning according to taste

Nutritional Values: Calories: 225, Fat: 4g, Carbs: 35g, Protein: 12g, Sugar: 5g, Sodium: 300 mg, Potassium: 840 mg, Cholesterol: 0 mg

Fish Chowder

Preparation Time: 20 min
Cooking Time: 45 min
Mode of Cooking: Stovetop
Servings: 6
Ingredients:

- 1 lb cod, cubed
- 2 potatoes, peeled and cubed
- 1 onion, diced
- 2 celery stalks, diced
- 3 C. fish stock
- 1 C. light cream
- 2 Tbsp butter
- 1 bay leaf
- Salt and pepper to taste
- 1/4 C. fresh parsley, chopped
- ½ C. corn kernels

Directions:

1. Melt butter in a large pot over medium heat
2. Add onion and celery, cook until soft
3. Add potatoes, fish stock, and bay leaf, bring to a boil and then simmer for 20 min
4. Add cod and corn, cook for an additional 10 min
5. Remove bay leaf, stir in cream, and heat through. Season with salt and pepper, garnish with parsley

Tips:

- Avoid boiling after adding cream to prevent curdling
- Ideal with oyster crackers or fresh bread
- For a thicker chowder, mash some of the potatoes in the soup

Nutritional Values: Calories: 290, Fat: 12g, Carbs: 27g, Protein: 19g, Sugar: 5g, Sodium: 410 mg, Potassium: 750 mg, Cholesterol: 55 mg

Chicken and Wild Rice Soup

Preparation Time: 20 min.
Cooking Time: 50 min.
Mode of Cooking: Simmering
Servings: 6
Ingredients:

- 1 lb chicken breast, cubed
- 1 cup wild rice
- 1 onion, finely chopped
- 2 carrots, diced
- 2 celery stalks, diced
- 4 cups low-sodium chicken broth
- 2 tsp dried thyme
- 1 tsp garlic powder
- Salt and pepper to taste
- 2 Tbsp olive oil

Directions:

1. Heat olive oil in a large pot over medium heat
2. Add onions, carrots, and celery, sauté until softened
3. Add chicken and cook until browned
4. Stir in garlic powder, thyme, salt, and pepper

5. Pour in chicken broth, bring to a boil
6. Add wild rice, reduce heat and simmer for 45 min. until rice is tender and chicken is cooked through

Tips:

- Garnish with fresh parsley for a pop of color and flavor
- Add a squeeze of lemon juice before serving to enhance flavors

Nutritional Values: Calories: 245, Fat: 6g, Carbs: 25g, Protein: 22g, Sugar: 3g, Sodium: 70 mg, Potassium: 340 mg, Cholesterol: 55 mg

Lentil and Spinach Soup

Preparation Time: 15 min.
Cooking Time: 35 min.
Mode of Cooking: Boiling
Servings: 4
Ingredients:

- 1 cup red lentils
- 4 cups vegetable stock
- 1 onion, chopped
- 2 garlic cloves, minced
- 1 tsp ground cumin
- 1 tsp curry powder
- 3 cups fresh spinach leaves
- 1 Tbsp olive oil
- Salt and pepper to taste

Directions:

1. Heat olive oil in a large saucepan over medium heat
2. Add onion and garlic, sauté until translucent
3. Stir in cumin and curry powder
4. Add lentils and vegetable stock, bring to a boil
5. Reduce heat and simmer for 25 min.
6. Stir in fresh spinach, cook until wilted
7. Season with salt and pepper

Tips:

- Serve with a dollop of yogurt and sprinkle of fresh cilantro for extra flavor and creaminess
- Consider adding a squeeze of lemon juice for a tangy finish

Nutritional Values: Calories: 190, Fat: 3g, Carbs: 30g, Protein: 12g, Sugar: 2g, Sodium: 300 mg, Potassium: 480 mg, Cholesterol: 0 mg

Chapter 9: Low-FODMAP Recipes

Embarking on a low-FODMAP diet can feel like navigating a labyrinth with twists and turns at every corner, especially for those of us managing diverticulitis. It's a diet that often requires a meticulous selection of foods—a challenge, yes, but one that brings with it a potential sigh of relief for your digestive system.

Low-FODMAP foods are essentially those that contain fewer sugars and fibers that ferment quickly during digestion, reducing instances of bloating, gas, and the pesky pain those of us with sensitive guts know all too well. However, embarking on this diet doesn't mean resigning yourself to bland meals or a monotonous plate. On the contrary, it opens a new door to culinary creativity—one that I am eager to guide you through in this chapter.

Imagine starting your day with a breakfast that's as satiating as it is soothing. Think of fluffy pancakes topped with a drizzle of maple syrup—not just any pancakes, but ones made from low-FODMAP friendly ingredients that won't leave you worrying about your next meal. Or envision a lunch that energizes rather than exhausts, with vibrant salads dressed in homemade, gut-friendly dressings.

For dinner, the low-FODMAP palette can be as rich and diverse as any other. From hearty, nourishing soups tailored to be gentle on your system to international dishes reimagined to suit your dietary needs—your culinary journey need not be restrictive.

This chapter not only offers recipes but also serves as your compass in the low-FODMAP world. It's about transforming the way we think about food and our condition, focusing not on limitations but on the vast array of possibilities. With each recipe, you're not just feeding your body; you're also nourishing your soul and taking control of diverticulitis, turning what could be a path of dietary restrictions into a journey of discovery and enjoyment. Here, let's explore how delectable, diverse, and satisfying low-FODMAP eating can be. Welcome to a world where your gut health is the priority, but your palate does not have to compromise.

9.1 Breakfast Options

Quinoa Porridge with Cinnamon and Pear

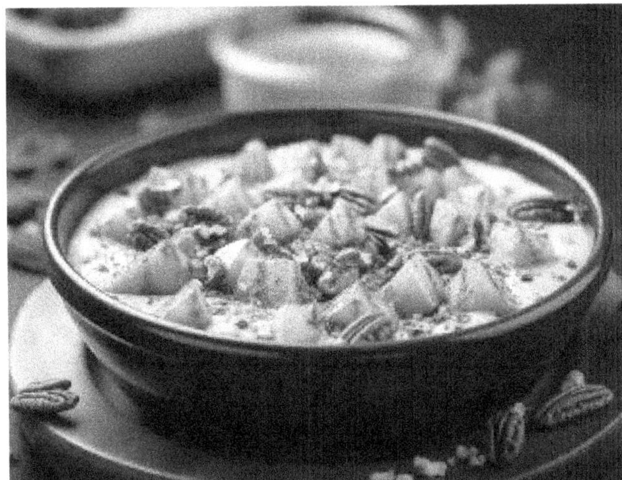

Preparation Time: 10 min
Cooking Time: 15 min
Mode of Cooking: Stovetop
Servings: 2

Ingredients:

- 1 cup quinoa, rinsed
- 2 cups water
- 1 ripe pear, peeled and diced
- ½ tsp cinnamon
- ¼ tsp salt
- 1 Tbsp maple syrup
- 2 Tbsp chopped pecans

Directions:

1. Combine quinoa and water in a medium saucepan and bring to a boil
2. Reduce heat to low and simmer covered until quinoa is tender and water is absorbed, about 15 minutes
3. Stir in cinnamon, salt, and pear, and cook for an additional 2 minutes

4. Remove from heat, drizzle with maple syrup, and garnish with chopped pecans

Tips:

- Serve with a dollop of lactose-free yogurt for added creaminess
- Experiment with different fruits such as bananas or apples for variety

Nutritional Values: Calories: 290, Fat: 5g, Carbs: 55g, Protein: 8g, Sugar: 12g, Sodium: 320 mg, Potassium: 400 mg, Cholesterol: 0 mg

Berry Smoothie Bowl

Preparation Time: 5 min
Cooking Time: none
Mode of Cooking: Blending
Servings: 1
Ingredients:

- 1 cup frozen mixed berries
- ½ banana
- 1 cup lactose-free vanilla yogurt
- ¼ cup gluten-free granola
- 1 Tbsp chia seeds
- 1 Tbsp coconut flakes, unsweetened

Directions:

1. Blend frozen berries, banana, and lactose-free yogurt until smooth
2. Pour into a bowl and top with gluten-free granola, chia seeds, and coconut flakes

Tips:

- Top with fresh berries for an extra burst of flavor and antioxidants
- Use a high-power blender for a smoother consistency

Nutritional Values: Calories: 380, Fat: 9g, Carbs: 62g, Protein: 13g, Sugar: 35g, Sodium: 85 mg, Potassium: 500 mg, Cholesterol: 5 mg

Savory Baked Eggs in Avocado

Preparation Time: 5 min
Cooking Time: 15 min
Mode of Cooking: Baking
Servings: 2
Ingredients:

- 1 large avocado, halved and pitted
- 2 eggs
- Salt to taste
- Black pepper to taste
- 2 Tbsp crumbled feta cheese
- 1 Tbsp chopped chives

Directions:

1. Preheat oven to 425°F (220°C)
2. Scoop out a bit more avocado from the center to enlarge the space for the egg
3. Crack an egg into each avocado half
4. Season with salt and pepper, and top with crumbled feta cheese
5. Place on a baking tray and bake until eggs are set, about 15 minutes
6. Garnish with chopped chives before serving

Tips:

- Use room temperature eggs for more even cooking
- Pair with a side of cooked spinach for a complete meal

Nutritional Values: Calories: 320, Fat: 27g, Carbs: 12g, Protein: 13g, Sugar: 1g, Sodium: 180 mg, Potassium: 800 mg, Cholesterol: 215 mg

Herbed Mushroom Omelet

Preparation Time: 10 min
Cooking Time: 10 min
Mode of Cooking: Stovetop
Servings: 1
Ingredients:

- 3 eggs, beaten
- ¼ cup chopped bell peppers
- ¼ cup diced low-FODMAP mushrooms (such as oyster or shiitake)
- 1 Tbsp olive oil
- Salt to taste

- Black pepper to taste
- 2 Tbsp grated Parmesan cheese
- 1 Tbsp chopped parsley

Directions:

1. Heat olive oil in a non-stick skillet over medium heat
2. Sauté bell peppers and mushrooms until soft, about 5 minutes
3. Pour beaten eggs over vegetables, season with salt and pepper, and cook until the edges start to lift from the pan
4. Sprinkle with Parmesan cheese and fold the omelet in half
5. Cook until cheese melts and eggs are fully set, about 5 minutes
6. Garnish with chopped parsley

Tips:

- Experiment with different herbs like basil or thyme for a new flavor profile
- Ensure a fluffy omelet by vigorously whisking the eggs before cooking

Nutritional Values: Calories: 400, Fat: 30g, Carbs: 6g, Protein: 24g, Sugar: 3g, Sodium: 470 mg, Potassium: 300 mg, Cholesterol: 390 mg

Quinoa Porridge with Cinnamon Apples

Preparation Time: 15 min
Cooking Time: 20 min
Mode of Cooking: Stovetop
Servings: 2
Ingredients:

- 1 C. quinoa, rinsed
- 2 C. lactose-free milk
- 1 tsp. cinnamon
- 1 Tbsp. maple syrup
- 1 medium apple, diced
- 1 pinch of salt

Directions:

1. Rinse quinoa thoroughly under cold water and drain
2. In a saucepan, combine quinoa, cinnamon, salt, and lactose-free milk, bring to a simmer over medium heat
3. Reduce heat and simmer for 15 min until quinoa is soft
4. Stir in maple syrup
5. In a separate pan, sauté the apple until tender and golden
6. Serve quinoa porridge topped with sautéed apples

Tips:

- Add a dollop of lactose-free yogurt for extra creaminess
- Garnish with a sprinkle of nutmeg for added flavor

Nutritional Values: Calories: 320, Fat: 5g, Carbs: 60g, Protein: 8g, Sugar: 15g, Sodium: 80 mg, Potassium: 480 mg, Cholesterol: 10 mg

9.2 Lunch and Dinner Recipes

Seared Chicken with Ginger-Spinach

Preparation Time: 15 min
Cooking Time: 10 min
Mode of Cooking: Pan-Frying
Servings: 2
Ingredients:

- 2 chicken breasts, boneless
- 1 Tbsp olive oil
- 1 tsp freshly grated ginger
- 2 cups fresh spinach
- ¼ tsp salt
- ¼ tsp black pepper
- 1 Tbsp garlic-infused oil
- 1 lemon, juiced

Directions:

1. Season chicken breasts with salt, pepper, and grated ginger
2. Heat olive oil in a skillet over medium heat and seared the chicken on both sides until

golden and cooked through, about 4-5 min. per side

3. Remove chicken and in the same pan, add garlic-infused oil, add spinach and sauté until wilted
4. Drizzle with lemon juice and serve with chicken

Tips:

- Use garlic-infused oil instead of garlic to keep it low-FODMAP
- Add a pinch of crushed red pepper flakes to spinach for a spicy kick

Nutritional Values: Calories: 295, Fat: 15g, Carbs: 4g, Protein: 34g, Sugar: 1g, Sodium: 380 mg, Potassium: 550 mg, Cholesterol: 95 mg

Grilled Fish with Lemon-Herb Quinoa

Preparation Time: 20 min
Cooking Time: 12 min
Mode of Cooking: Grilling
Servings: 2
Ingredients:

- 2 fish fillets, firm white fish such as cod or tilapia
- 1 Tbsp olive oil
- ½ tsp salt
- ½ tsp pepper
- 1 cup quinoa
- 1 Tbsp lemon zest
- 2 Tbsp lemon juice
- 1 Tbsp chopped fresh parsley
- 1 Tbsp chopped fresh basil
- 1 Tbsp garlic-infused oil

Directions:

1. Rinse quinoa thoroughly and cook according to package instructions
2. Season fish fillets with salt and pepper and brush with olive oil
3. Grill over medium-high heat for 5-6 min on each side
4. Mix cooked quinoa with lemon zest, lemon juice, parsley, basil, and garlic-infused oil to serve alongside fish

Tips:

- Opt for fresh herbs to enhance flavor without adding FODMAPs
- Lemon zest adds a fresh burst of flavor without added sugars

Nutritional Values: Calories: 410, Fat: 14g, Carbs: 38g, Protein: 35g, Sugar: 1g, Sodium: 560 mg, Potassium: 840 mg, Cholesterol: 85 mg

Low-FODMAP Meatloaf

Preparation Time: 15 min
Cooking Time: 1 hr
Mode of Cooking: Baking
Servings: 4
Ingredients:

- 1 lb ground turkey
- 2 Tbsp chives, chopped
- ¼ cup gluten-free breadcrumbs
- ¼ cup lactose-free milk
- 1 egg
- 1 tsp salt
- ½ tsp pepper
- 2 Tbsp tomato paste
- 1 Tbsp Worcestershire sauce
- 1 Tbsp garlic-infused oil for greasing

Directions:

1. Mix ground turkey, chives, breadcrumbs, lactose-free milk, egg, salt, and pepper in a bowl
2. Combine tomato paste and Worcestershire sauce in a separate bowl
3. Mix both mixtures together properly
4. Press into a loaf pan greased with garlic-infused oil
5. Bake at 375°F (190°C) for 1 hr or until cooked through

Tips:

- Use gluten-free breadcrumbs to avoid gluten and maintain low FODMAP
- You can replace tomato paste with pureed red peppers, if sensitive to tomatoes

Nutritional Values: Calories: 330, Fat: 17g, Carbs: 14g, Protein: 28g, Sugar: 5g, Sodium: 870 mg, Potassium: 470 mg, Cholesterol: 140 mg

Seared Chicken with Garlic Spinach

Preparation Time: 10 min
Cooking Time: 15 min
Mode of Cooking: Sautéing
Servings: 2
Ingredients:

- 2 boneless, skinless chicken breasts
- 1 Tbsp olive oil
- 2 cups fresh spinach
- 1 tsp garlic-infused oil
- Salt and pepper to taste
- Lemon wedges for serving

Directions:

1. Season chicken breasts with salt and pepper
2. Heat olive oil in a skillet over medium-high heat
3. Add chicken to the skillet and sear for 6-7 min on each side or until golden and cooked through
4. Remove chicken and set aside
5. In the same skillet, add garlic-infused oil and spinach
6. Sauté until spinach is wilted
7. Serve chicken topped with sautéed spinach and lemon wedges

Tips:

- Use garlic-infused oil instead of garlic for low-FODMAP compliance
- Serve with a side of mashed potatoes or rice for a fuller meal

Nutritional Values: Calories: 295, Fat: 15g, Carbs: 3g, Protein: 35g, Sugar: 0g, Sodium: 70 mg, Potassium: 450 mg, Cholesterol: 95 mg

Grilled Fish with Herbed Quinoa

Preparation Time: 15 min
Cooking Time: 12 min
Mode of Cooking: Grilling
Servings: 2
Ingredients:

- 2 fish fillets (such as tilapia or cod)
- 1 Tbsp olive oil
- 1 cup quinoa
- 2 cups FODMAP-friendly vegetable stock
- 1 Tbsp chopped fresh parsley
- 1 Tbsp chopped fresh basil
- 1 lemon, sliced
- Salt and pepper to taste

Directions:

1. Rinse quinoa under cold water
2. Cook quinoa in FODMAP-friendly vegetable stock according to package instructions
3. Brush fish fillets with olive oil and season with salt and pepper
4. Grill fillets over medium heat for about 6 min on each side or until fully cooked and flaky
5. Mix cooked quinoa with fresh parsley, basil, and juice from lemon slices
6. Serve grilled fish over herbed quinoa

Tips:

- Opt for herbs like parsley and basil to add flavor without adding FODMAPs
- Quinoa is a great source of protein and is low in FODMAPs when cooked properly
- Adding lemon juice not only enhances taste but also aids in digestion

Nutritional Values: Calories: 410, Fat: 12g, Carbs: 49g, Protein: 32g, Sugar: 2g, Sodium: 85 mg, Potassium: 770 mg, Cholesterol: 85 mg

9.3 Snacks and Desserts

Coconut Macaroons Delight

Preparation Time: 15 min
Cooking Time: 25 min
Mode of Cooking: Baking
Servings: 24
Ingredients:

- 1-1/2 cups unsweetened shredded coconut
- 3 large egg whites
- 1/4 cup maple syrup
- 1 tsp pure vanilla extract
- 1/4 tsp sea salt

Directions:

1. Whisk egg whites, maple syrup, vanilla extract, and salt in a bowl until fully combined
2. Fold in shredded coconut until mixture is moistened and sticks together
3. Using a scoop, place mounds of coconut mixture on a parchment-lined baking tray, ensuring they are spaced apart
4. Bake in a preheated oven at 325°F (163°C) until the edges are golden brown
5. Let cool on the tray for 10 min before transferring to a wire rack

Tips:

- Use a silicone mat for easier removal and to prevent sticking
- Store in an airtight container to maintain freshness

Nutritional Values: Calories: 60, Fat: 4.5g, Carbs: 4g, Protein: 1g, Sugar: 3g, Sodium: 20 mg, Potassium: 10 mg, Cholesterol: 0 mg

Low-FODMAP Trail Mix

Preparation Time: 10 min
Cooking Time: none
Mode of Cooking: No Cooking
Servings: 8
Ingredients:

- 1 cup toasted pumpkin seeds
- 1/2 cup roasted pecans
- 1/2 cup dried cranberries, unsweetened and low-FODMAP certified
- 1/4 cup toasted coconut flakes

Directions:

1. Combine toasted pumpkin seeds, roasted pecans, dried cranberries, and toasted coconut flakes in a large bowl
2. Mix thoroughly to distribute the flavors evenly
3. Store in an airtight container at room temperature

Tips:

- Opt to use seeds and nuts according to personal tolerance levels
- Add a pinch of salt to enhance flavors if desired

Nutritional Values: Calories: 200, Fat: 15g, Carbs: 12g, Protein: 5g, Sugar: 5g, Sodium: 5 mg, Potassium: 150 mg, Cholesterol: 0 mg

Refreshing Fruit Sorbet

Preparation Time: 20 min
Cooking Time: 2 hr
Mode of Cooking: Freezing
Servings: 6
Ingredients:

- 2 cups frozen strawberries
- 1/2 cup frozen blueberries
- 1/4 cup maple syrup
- 2 Tbsp fresh orange juice
- 1 tsp fresh lemon juice

Directions:

1. Combine frozen strawberries, blueberries, maple syrup, orange juice, and lemon juice in a blender or food processor
2. Blend until smooth and creamy
3. Pour mixture into a freezable container and freeze for at least 2 hr or until firm
4. Scoop and serve immediately

Tips:

- For smoother texture, stir every 30 min during the freezing process
- Serve immediately after scooping for best flavor and consistency
- Add mint leaves for garnish and a touch of freshness

Nutritional Values: Calories: 90, Fat: 0.3g, Carbs: 22g, Protein: 1g, Sugar: 18g, Sodium: 3 mg, Potassium: 85 mg, Cholesterol: 0 mg

Coconut Lemon Zest Macaroons

Preparation Time: 15 min
Cooking Time: 20 min
Mode of Cooking: Baking
Servings: 24
Ingredients:

- 2 cups fine shredded coconut, unsweetened
- ½ cup granulated cane sugar
- 3 Tbsp coconut flour
- ¼ tsp salt
- 3 large egg whites
- 1 Tbsp lemon zest
- 1 tsp vanilla extract

Directions:

1. Preheat oven to 325°F (163°C)
2. Mix coconut, sugar, coconut flour, and salt in a bowl
3. In a separate bowl, beat egg whites until peaks form
4. Fold in lemon zest and vanilla into egg whites
5. Gently fold the egg white mixture into the dry ingredients
6. Scoop tablespoon-sized mounds onto a baking sheet lined with parchment paper
7. Bake until golden, approximately 20 min

Tips:

- Allow macaroons to cool on the baking sheet for easier handling
- Store in an airtight container to preserve freshness

Nutritional Values: Calories: 100, Fat: 5g, Carbs: 12g, Protein: 1g, Sugar: 10g, Sodium: 50 mg, Potassium: 60 mg, Cholesterol: 0 mg

Low-FODMAP Trail Mix

Preparation Time: 10 min
Cooking Time: none
Mode of Cooking: No Cooking
Servings: 10
Ingredients:

- ½ cup roasted pumpkin seeds, unsalted
- ½ cup roasted pecans
- ¼ cup dried cranberries, sugar-free
- ¼ cup banana chips, no sugar added
- 1 tsp cinnamon powder
- 1 pinch sea salt

Directions:

1. Mix all ingredients together in a large bowl until evenly distributed

Tips:

- Store in a cool, dry place in an airtight container to maintain crunchiness and freshness
- For added flavor, sprinkle mix with a touch of low-FODMAP maple or rice syrup

Nutritional Values: Calories: 150, Fat: 10g, Carbs: 13g, Protein: 3g, Sugar: 7g, Sodium: 5 mg, Potassium: 125 mg, Cholesterol: 0 mg

Chapter 10: High-Fiber Recipes

Welcome to a pivotal chapter in our journey towards revitalizing gut health through the power of nutrition. If you've been following along, you already know about the gentle, soothing ways we can nurture our abdominal health. Now, let's focus on the robust world of high-fiber recipes, especially curated to enhance digestive function and foster recovery from the grips of diverticulitis.

You might wonder why fiber warrants dedicated attention in our dietary arsenal. Fiber is not just any component of our meals; it's akin to the diligent worker that helps keep our digestive system active and efficient. Its role extends beyond sheer function; it's about creating a thriving environment in our gut. High-fiber foods act like a scrub, compassionately and gently cleansing our intestinal walls, ensuring they remain free from inflammation and reducing the risks associated with diverticulitis flare-ups.

As we explore these recipes, we engage with more than the nutritional value of fiber; we embrace a lifestyle that nourishes our bodies while providing them the strength to heal and defend against future ailments. The recipes in this chapter are designed not only to excite your palate but also to blend seamlessly into your busy life. We recognize the challenges of balancing work, family, and health, and aim to lighten that load with meals that are as quick as they are beneficial.

Think of each dish not just as sustenance but as a step toward better health—a comforting bowl of oatmeal in the morning, a vibrant bean salad at lunch, or a hearty vegetable stew for dinner. These dishes promise to deliver not only the needed nutrients but also the confidence and peace of mind that come from knowing you're doing right by your body.

As you turn these pages, remember that each recipe is more than just ingredients and instructions; they are a testament to a lifestyle choice, a companion in your journey to recovery and long-term health management. Let's redesign your kitchen into a haven of health, one high-fiber meal at a time.

10.1 Breakfast Choices

Chia & Berry Sunrise Smoothie

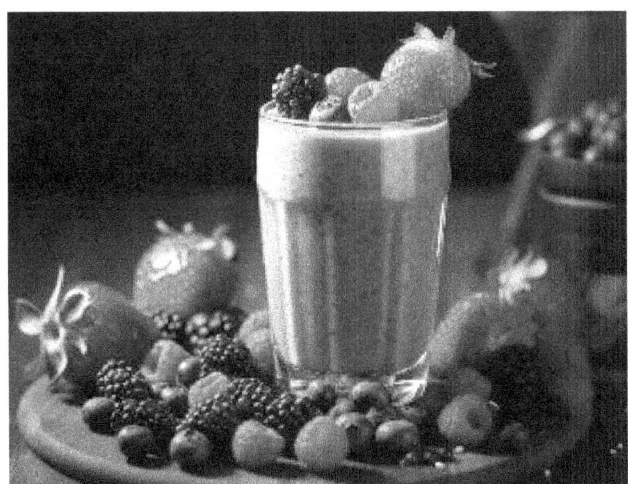

Preparation Time: 10 min
Cooking Time: none
Mode of Cooking: Blending
Servings: 2

Ingredients:

- 1 cup unsweetened almond milk
- 1/3 cup chia seeds
- 1 cup mixed berries, fresh or frozen
- 1 banana, sliced
- 1 Tbsp ground flaxseed
- 1 Tbsp honey or maple syrup
- 1/2 tsp vanilla extract

Directions:

1. Combine almond milk and chia seeds and let sit for 5 min to allow chia seeds to swell
2. Add swollen chia mixture, mixed berries, banana, ground flaxseed, honey, and vanilla extract to blender
3. Blend on high until smooth

Tips:

- Add a scoop of protein powder for an extra boost
- Use frozen berries for a thicker consistency
- Substitute honey with agave syrup for a vegan option

Nutritional Values: Calories: 295, Fat: 9g, Carbs: 50g, Protein: 8g, Sugar: 20g, Sodium: 55 mg, Potassium: 411 mg, Cholesterol: 0 mg

HIGH-FIBER BLUEBERRY PANCAKES

Preparation Time: 15 min
Cooking Time: 10 min
Mode of Cooking: Frying
Servings: 4
Ingredients:

- 1 cup whole wheat flour
- 1/2 cup rolled oats
- 1/4 cup ground flaxseed
- 2 tsp baking powder
- 1/2 tsp salt
- 1 tsp cinnamon
- 1 cup low-fat milk
- 2 eggs
- 1 Tbsp olive oil
- 1 Tbsp honey
- 1 cup fresh blueberries

Directions:

1. Mix whole wheat flour, rolled oats, ground flaxseed, baking powder, salt, and cinnamon in a bowl
2. In a separate bowl, whisk low-fat milk, eggs, olive oil, and honey
3. Combine wet and dry ingredients until just mixed; fold in blueberries
4. Heat a non-stick skillet over medium heat; pour 1/4 cup batter for each pancake; cook until bubbles form on top, then flip and cook until golden

Tips:

- Serve with extra fresh blueberries and a drizzle of maple syrup for enhanced flavor
- Use almond milk for a dairy-free version
- Add a dollop of Greek yogurt on top for additional protein

Nutritional Values: Calories: 254, Fat: 8g, Carbs: 38g, Protein: 9g, Sugar: 12g, Sodium: 300 mg, Potassium: 222 mg, Cholesterol: 93 mg

TROPICAL FIBER MUFFINS

Preparation Time: 20 min
Cooking Time: 25 min
Mode of Cooking: Baking
Servings: 12
Ingredients:

- 1 1/2 cups oat bran
- 1 cup whole wheat flour
- 1/2 cup brown sugar
- 2 tsp baking soda
- 1 tsp baking powder
- 1/2 tsp salt
- 1 cup chopped pineapple
- 1/2 cup shredded coconut
- 1/2 cup raisins
- 1/2 cup chopped nuts
- 1 egg
- 1 cup buttermilk
- 1/4 cup vegetable oil
- 1 tsp vanilla extract

Directions:

1. Mix oat bran, whole wheat flour, brown sugar, baking soda, baking powder, and salt in a large bowl
2. Add pineapple, coconut, raisins, and nuts to dry ingredients
3. In another bowl, whisk egg, buttermilk, vegetable oil, and vanilla extract
4. Combine wet and dry ingredients until just moistened

5. Spoon into muffin tins lined with paper cups, filling each 3/4 full
6. Bake in a preheated oven at 375°F (190°C) until a toothpick inserted comes out clean

Tips:

- Use apple sauce instead of vegetable oil for a lower-fat option
- Add a sprinkle of raw sugar on top before baking for a crunchy top
- Experiment with different tropical fruits like mango or papaya for variety

Nutritional Values: Calories: 279, Fat: 9g, Carbs: 45g, Protein: 6g, Sugar: 20g, Sodium: 407 mg, Potassium: 263 mg, Cholesterol: 18 mg

Apple & Cinnamon Bran Porridge

Preparation Time: 5 min
Cooking Time: 15 min
Mode of Cooking: Cooking
Servings: 2
Ingredients:

- 1 cup bran flakes
- 2 cups water
- 1 apple, peeled and diced
- 1/2 tsp cinnamon
- 1 Tbsp honey
- 2 Tbsp chopped walnuts
- 1/2 cup low-fat milk

Directions:

1. Combine bran flakes and water in a saucepan and bring to a boil
2. Reduce heat to low; add diced apple and simmer for 10 min
3. Stir in cinnamon, honey, and chopped walnuts; continue to cook for another 5 min
4. Serve hot with a splash of low-fat milk

Tips:

- Sprinkle with additional cinnamon if desired for extra flavor
- Sweeten with maple syrup instead of honey if preferred
- Top with a dollop of Greek yogurt for creaminess and protein

Nutritional Values: Calories: 210, Fat: 4g, Carbs: 40g, Protein: 5g, Sugar: 20g, Sodium: 190 mg, Potassium: 220 mg, Cholesterol: 1 mg

Quinoa and Oat Blueberry Pancakes

Preparation Time: 15 min
Cooking Time: 10 min
Mode of Cooking: Pan Frying
Servings: 4
Ingredients:

- 1 C. cooked quinoa
- 1 C. rolled oats
- 2 tsp baking powder
- ½ tsp salt
- 1 C. blueberries, fresh
- 2 large eggs
- 1 C. almond milk
- 2 Tbsp maple syrup
- 1 Tbsp coconut oil, melted
- ½ tsp vanilla extract

Directions:

1. Combine quinoa, oats, baking powder, and salt in a bowl
2. In a separate bowl, whisk eggs, almond milk, maple syrup, melted coconut oil, and vanilla extract until smooth
3. Combine wet and dry ingredients and fold in blueberries gently
4. Heat a non-stick skillet over medium heat and pour ¼ C. batter for each pancake, cook until bubbles form on top, then flip and cook until golden brown

Tips:

- Avoid overmixing the batter to keep pancakes fluffy

- Serve with extra blueberries and a drizzle of honey if desired

Nutritional Values: Calories: 290, Fat: 8g, Carbs: 46g, Protein: 8g, Sugar: 12g, Sodium: 300 mg, Potassium: 200 mg, Cholesterol: 95 mg

10.2 Fiber-Rich Mains

Quinoa & Chard Stuffed Peppers

Preparation Time: 20 min
Cooking Time: 45 min
Mode of Cooking: Baking
Servings: 4
Ingredients:

- 1 cup quinoa, cooked
- 4 large bell peppers, halved and seeded
- 1 bunch Swiss chard, chopped finely
- 1 onion, diced
- 2 cloves garlic, minced
- 1 tsp cumin
- 1 tsp coriander
- 1/2 cup feta cheese, crumbled
- 1/4 cup pine nuts, toasted
- 1 Tbsp olive oil
- Salt and pepper to taste

Directions:

1. Preheat oven to 375°F (190°C)
2. In a skillet, heat olive oil and sauté onion and garlic until translucent
3. Add Swiss chard, cumin, and coriander, cooking until chard is wilted
4. Remove from heat and stir in cooked quinoa, feta, and pine nuts
5. Fill each pepper half with the quinoa mixture and place in a baking dish
6. Cover with foil and bake for 35 minutes, then remove foil and bake for another 10 minutes

Tips:

- Serve with a dollop of Greek yogurt for added creaminess
- Sprinkle with fresh herbs like parsley or cilantro for extra flavor

Nutritional Values: Calories: 295, Fat: 9g, Carbs: 44g, Protein: 12g, Sugar: 6g, Sodium: 310 mg, Potassium: 770 mg, Cholesterol: 15 mg

Barley and Mushroom Pilaf

Preparation Time: 15 min
Cooking Time: 30 min
Mode of Cooking: Simmering
Servings: 6
Ingredients:

- 1 cup barley, rinsed
- 3 cups mushroom broth
- 1 cup mixed mushrooms, sliced
- 1 onion, chopped
- 2 Tbsp olive oil
- 1 Tbsp fresh thyme leaves
- Salt and pepper to taste

Directions:

1. In a large saucepan, heat olive oil and sauté onions until translucent
2. Add mushrooms and cook until browned
3. Stir in barley and toast slightly before adding mushroom broth
4. Bring to a boil, then reduce to a simmer and cover for 30 minutes or until barley is tender

Tips:

- This dish pairs beautifully with a side of steamed green beans
- Add a splash of white wine to the mushrooms for added depth

Nutritional Values: Calories: 180, Fat: 7g, Carbs: 27g, Protein: 4g, Sugar: 2g, Sodium: 55 mg, Potonium: 250 mg, Cholesterol: 0 mg

Black Bean Tacos

Preparation Time: 15 min
Cooking Time: 10 min
Mode of Cooking: Sautéing
Servings: 6
Ingredients:

- 12 small corn tortillas
- 2 cups black beans, cooked
- 1 avocado, diced
- 1 cup cabbage, shredded
- 1 small red onion, thinly sliced
- 2 Tbsp cilantro, chopped
- 1 lime, juiced
- 2 Tbsp olive oil
- 1 tsp smoked paprika
- Salt and pepper to taste

Directions:

1. Heat olive oil in a pan, add black beans and smoked paprika, and cook until warm
2. Warm tortillas in a separate skillet or microwave
3. Assemble tacos: spoon black beans into tortillas, top with cabbage, onion, avocado, cilantro, and drizzle with lime juice

Tips:

- Experiment with different toppings like radishes or pickled jalapeños for a spicy kick
- For extra protein, add grilled chicken or fish

Nutritional Values: Calories: 215, Fat: 8g, Carbs: 33g, Protein: 7g, Sugar: 2g, Sodium: 250 mg, Potassium: 450 mg, Cholesterol: 0 mg

Lentil and Spinach Stew

Preparation Time: 10 min
Cooking Time: 35 min
Mode of Cooking: Simmering
Servings: 4
Ingredients:

- 1 cup lentils, rinsed
- 4 cups vegetable broth
- 1 onion, diced
- 2 carrots, diced
- 2 stalks celery, diced
- 2 cloves garlic, minced
- 2 cups spinach leaves
- 1 tsp turmeric
- 1 tsp cumin
- 2 Tbsp olive oil
- Salt and pepper to taste

Directions:

1. In a large pot, heat olive oil over medium heat
2. Add onions, carrots, celery, and garlic, sautéing until onions are translucent
3. Add lentils, turmeric, cumin, and vegetable broth, bringing to a boil then simmering for 30 minutes
4. Stir in spinach just before serving and cook until wilted

Tips:

- Serve with a sprinkle of lemon juice for a refreshing twist
- Accompany with whole-grain bread for a hearty meal

Nutritional Values: Calories: 240, Fat: 5g, Carbs: 38g, Protein: 12g, Sugar: 4g, Sodium: 300 mg, Potassium: 700 mg, Cholesterol: 0 mg

Black Bean and Quinoa Tacos

Preparation Time: 15 min
Cooking Time: 20 min
Mode of Cooking: Stovetop
Servings: 4
Ingredients:

- 1 C. quinoa, rinsed
- 2 C. vegetable broth
- 1 Tbsp olive oil
- 1 onion, finely chopped
- 2 garlic cloves, minced
- 1 tsp cumin

- 1 tsp paprika
- 1 can black beans, drained and rinsed
- 8 small corn tortillas
- 1 avocado, diced
- ½ C. fresh cilantro, chopped
- 1 lime, cut into wedges

Directions:

1. Heat olive oil in a skillet on medium heat. Sauté onion and garlic until translucent
2. Stir in cumin, paprika, and quinoa, then pour in vegetable broth. Bring to a boil, then cover and reduce heat to simmer for 15 min until quinoa is cooked
3. Stir in black beans and heat through
4. Warm tortillas and assemble tacos with quinoa-bean mixture, top with avocado, cilantro, and a squeeze of lime

Tips:

- Serve with a dollop of Greek yogurt for creaminess
- Customize with your favorite salsa for extra flavor

Nutritional Values: Calories: 290, Fat: 8g, Carbs: 45g, Protein: 11g, Sugar: 3g, Sodium: 250 mg, Potassium: 672 mg, Cholesterol: 0 mg

10.3 Healthy Desserts

Fiber-Boosted Chia Pudding

Preparation Time: 15 min
Cooking Time: none
Mode of Cooking: No Cooking
Servings: 4
Ingredients:

- 1 cup unsweetened almond milk
- ¼ cup chia seeds
- 1 Tbsp maple syrup
- ½ tsp vanilla extract
- ¼ tsp ground cinnamon
- ½ cup fresh blueberries
- ¼ cup sliced strawberries

Directions:

1. Combine almond milk, chia seeds, maple syrup, vanilla extract, and cinnamon in a bowl
2. Stir well until the chia seeds are evenly distributed
3. Refrigerate for at least 4 hours or overnight to allow the chia seeds to swell and thicken the mixture
4. Top with fresh blueberries and sliced strawberries before serving

Tips:

- Serve with a dollop of Greek yogurt for added protein
- Customize with different berries or fruits depending on season and preference

Nutritional Values: Calories: 130, Fat: 6g, Carbs: 18g, Protein: 4g, Sugar: 8g, Sodium: 45 mg, Potassium: 90 mg, Cholesterol: 0 mg

Quinoa Apple Crisp

Preparation Time: 20 min
Cooking Time: 45 min
Mode of Cooking: Baking
Servings: 6
Ingredients:

- 1 cup quinoa, rinsed and drained
- 4 medium-sized apples, peeled, cored, and sliced
- 1/3 cup raisins
- 1 tsp cinnamon
- ½ tsp nutmeg
- ¼ cup walnuts, chopped
- 2 Tbsp coconut oil, melted
- 3 Tbsp honey

Directions:

1. Preheat oven to 375°F (190°C)
2. In a mixing bowl, combine quinoa, cinnamon, nutmeg, and walnuts

3. In a separate bowl, toss the apple slices with raisins and honey
4. Place the apple mixture in a baking dish
5. Sprinkle the quinoa mixture on top
6. Drizzle with melted coconut oil
7. Bake in the preheated oven for about 45 min or until the topping is golden and crisp

Tips:

- Best served warm
- Pair with low-fat vanilla ice cream or Greek yogurt for a creamy texture

Nutritional Values: Calories: 210, Fat: 8g, Carbs: 34g, Protein: 4g, Sugar: 19g, Sodium: 10 mg, Potassium: 276 mg, Cholesterol: 0 mg

Whole Wheat Banana Muffins

Preparation Time: 15 min
Cooking Time: 20 min
Mode of Cooking: Baking
Servings: 12
Ingredients:

- 2 cups whole wheat flour
- 1 tsp baking powder
- ½ tsp baking soda
- ½ tsp salt
- 4 ripe bananas, mashed
- ⅓ cup melted coconut oil
- ½ cup honey
- 2 eggs
- 1 tsp vanilla extract
- ½ cup walnuts, chopped

Directions:

1. Preheat oven to 375°F (190°C)
2. In a large bowl, mix together whole wheat flour, baking powder, baking soda, and salt
3. In another bowl, combine mashed bananas, coconut oil, honey, eggs, and vanilla extract
4. Add the wet ingredients to the dry ingredients and stir until just combined
5. Fold in chopped walnuts
6. Spoon the batter into a muffin tin lined with paper liners
7. Bake for about 20 min or until a toothpick inserted into the center of a muffin comes out clean

Tips:

- Store in an airtight container to retain freshness
- These muffins can be frozen for up to one month for quick breakfast options

Nutritional Values: Calories: 220, Fat: 10g, Carbs: 30g, Protein: 5g, Sugar: 14g, Sodium: 200 mg, Potassium: 240 mg, Cholesterol: 31 mg

Baked Cinnamon Stuffed Apples

Preparation Time: 15 min
Cooking Time: 30 min
Mode of Cooking: Baking
Servings: 6
Ingredients:

- 6 large apples, cored
- ½ cup oats
- ¼ cup almonds, chopped
- ¼ cup dried cranberries
- ¼ cup brown sugar
- 1 tsp cinnamon
- ¼ tsp nutmeg
- 3 Tbsp butter, cubed
- ¼ cup apple cider

Directions:

1. Preheat oven to 350°F (175°C)
2. Mix oats, almonds, dried cranberries, brown sugar, cinnamon, and nutmeg in a bowl
3. Stuff each cored apple with the oat mixture
4. Top each with a cube of butter
5. Pour apple cider into the baking dish around the apples
6. Cover with aluminum foil and bake for 20 min

7. Uncover and bake for an additional 10 min or until the apples are soft and the filling is bubbly

Tips:

- Ideal when served warm
- Try drizzling with a little honey or maple syrup for extra sweetness

Nutritional Values: Calories: 290, Fat: 12g, Carbs: 48g, Protein: 3g, Sugar: 35g, Sodium: 60 mg, Potassium: 200 mg, Cholesterol: 15 mg

Fiber-Rich Chia & Fig Pudding

Preparation Time: 15 min
Cooking Time: none
Mode of Cooking: No Cooking
Servings: 6
Ingredients:

- 2 C. almond milk
- 6 Tbsp chia seeds
- 1 tsp vanilla extract
- 3 Tbsp maple syrup
- 6 dried figs, diced
- 1/4 C. crushed pistachios

Directions:

1. Combine almond milk, chia seeds, vanilla extract, and maple syrup in a bowl
2. Stir thoroughly until the mixture begins to thicken
3. Fold in diced figs and refrigerate overnight
4. Serve chilled topped with crushed pistachios

Tips:

- Add a dollop of Greek yogurt for protein
- Sweeten with additional maple syrup if desired
- Figs can be substituted with dates for a different flavor

Nutritional Values: Calories: 180, Fat: 9g, Carbs: 24g, Protein: 5g, Sugar: 15g, Sodium: 30 mg, Potassium: 200 mg, Cholesterol: 0 mg

CHAPTER 11: RECOVERY PHASE RECIPES

Embarking on the recovery phase of your journey with diverticulitis marks a significant milestone. This transition is not just about healing—it's about gently reintroducing your body to the broader spectrum of foods and celebrating each small victory along the way. Imagine each meal as a step towards rebuilding your strength and resilience, where your gut is nurtured with every bite, leading you closer to a revitalized sense of well-being.

In this chapter, we focus on recipes that are designed to be both soothing and nourishing, tailored specifically to meet the needs of your digestive system as it recuperates. Picture this: It's early morning, and you are starting your day with a bowl of oat porridge simmered gently with almond milk—topped with a drizzle of honey and sliced bananas. It's not just a meal; it's a moment of peace for your healing intestines.

As your day progresses, the simplicity continues with meals that are crafted to support, not strain, your recovery. For lunch, visualize a pureed carrot soup, warm and velvety, infused with ginger to calm your digestion, and a sprinkle of thyme for a touch of freshness. These dishes aren't just made; they are curated with love for both taste and therapeutic value, ensuring they are as pleasing to the palate as they are comforting to the stomach.

Dinner might feature a baked salmon seasoned with dill and served alongside mashed pumpkin—foods chosen for their ease of digestion and nutrient density. These meals are your companions in healing, designed to reassure and nurture you back to health without any discomfort.

Through this careful selection of ingredients and preparation techniques, this chapter aims to provide you with a culinary toolkit that makes the recovery phase not only manageable but enjoyable. Embrace these recipes as your allies in health, knowing that each dish brings you closer to resuming your vibrant life, free from the shadows of discomfort that once loomed. So, let's take these steps together, one recipe at a time, towards a healthier, happier you.

11.1 GENTLE AND NUTRITIOUS

BLENDED ZUCCHINI BASIL SOUP

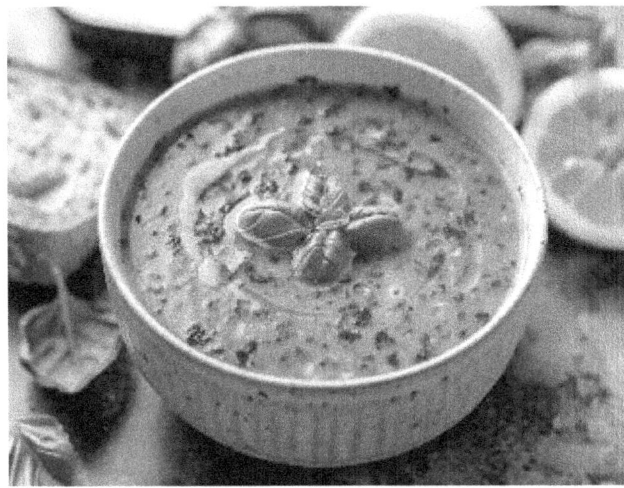

Preparation Time: 15 min
Cooking Time: 25 min
Mode of Cooking: Stovetop
Servings: 4

Ingredients:

- 2 medium zucchinis, roughly chopped
- 1 small onion, diced
- 2 cloves garlic, minced
- 4 cups low-sodium vegetable broth
- ½ cup fresh basil leaves
- 1 Tbsp olive oil
- Salt and pepper to taste
- 1 tsp lemon juice

Directions:

1. Heat olive oil in a large pot over medium heat
2. Add onion and garlic, sauté until translucent
3. Add chopped zucchini and cook for about 5 min

4. Pour in the vegetable broth and bring to a boil
5. Reduce heat and simmer for 20 min
6. Remove from heat, add basil and lemon juice
7. Blend the soup using an immersion blender until smooth

Tips:

- Consider garnishing with a dollop of Greek yogurt for added creaminess
- Serve warm or chilled depending on preference

Nutritional Values: Calories: 90, Fat: 4g, Carbs: 12g, Protein: 2g, Sugar: 7g, Sodium: 70mg, Potassium: 470mg, Cholesterol: 0mg

Softly Cooked Rice and Steamed Veggies

Preparation Time: 10 min
Cooking Time: 25 min
Mode of Cooking: Stovetop
Servings: 4
Ingredients:

- 1 cup jasmine rice
- 2 cups water
- 1 cup carrots, diced
- 1 cup zucchini, sliced
- 1 cup broccoli florets
- Salt to taste
- 1 Tbsp olive oil

Directions:

1. Rinse jasmine rice until water runs clear
2. In a saucepan, combine rice and water, bring to a boil
3. Reduce heat to low, cover and simmer for 15 min
4. In a separate steamer, steam carrots, zucchini, and broccoli until tender, about 10 min
5. Fluff rice with a fork and mix in steamed vegetables and olive oil

Tips:

- Add a sprinkle of fresh chopped parsley or dill for an extra touch of flavor
- Ensure rice is thoroughly cooked to a soft texture to make it easier to digest

Nutritional Values: Calories: 210, Fat: 4.5g, Carbs: 39g, Protein: 5g, Sugar: 3g, Sodium: 30mg, Potassium: 300mg, Cholesterol: 0mg

Ginger Poached Chicken

Preparation Time: 10 min
Cooking Time: 30 min
Mode of Cooking: Stovetop
Servings: 4
Ingredients:

- 4 boneless, skinless chicken breasts
- 4 cups chicken broth, low sodium
- 1 inch ginger, sliced
- 1 stalk lemongrass, bruised
- Salt to taste
- 2 Tbsp cilantro, chopped

Directions:

1. Fill a pot with chicken broth, ginger, and lemongrass
2. Bring to a gentle boil
3. Add chicken breasts to the pot and ensure they are submerged
4. Turn heat to low and poach chicken for about 20-25 min until fully cooked
5. Remove chicken, slice and garnish with cilantro

Tips:

- Serve with a side of steamed bok choy or spinach to incorporate more greens
- Poaching in ginger and lemongrass can enhance digestion and soothe the gut

Nutritional Values: Calories: 165, Fat: 3g, Carbs: 0g, Protein: 31g, Sugar: 0g, Sodium: 110mg, Potassium: 330mg, Cholesterol: 75mg

Carrot Ginger Puree

Preparation Time: 10 min
Cooking Time: 20 min
Mode of Cooking: Stovetop
Servings: 4
Ingredients:

- 1 lb carrots, peeled and chopped
- 2 tsp grated ginger
- 1 clove garlic, minced
- 1 Tbsp coconut oil
- ½ cup coconut milk
- Salt and pepper to taste

Directions:

1. In a medium saucepan, heat coconut oil over medium heat
2. Add minced garlic and grated ginger, sauté for 2 min
3. Add chopped carrots and cook for another 3 min
4. Add enough water to just cover the carrots, bring to a boil, then simmer until carrots are tender, about 15 min
5. Drain carrots, reserve liquid
6. Blend carrots and coconut milk, adding reserved liquid as needed to achieve desired consistency

Tips:

- For increased nutrient absorption add a pinch of turmeric
- This creamy puree can also be used as a base for soups or sauces

Nutritional Values: Calories: 130, Fat: 7g, Carbs: 15g, Protein: 2g, Sugar: 6g, Sodium: 85mg, Potassium: 390mg, Cholesterol: 0mg

Soft Jasmine Rice with Steamed Carrots and Zucchini

Preparation Time: 5 min
Cooking Time: 25 min
Mode of Cooking: Stovetop
Servings: 4
Ingredients:

- 1 cup jasmine rice, rinsed
- 2 cups water
- 1/2 tsp salt
- 1 cup carrots, peeled and sliced thinly
- 1 cup zucchini, sliced thinly
- 1 Tbsp olive oil

Directions:

1. Combine rinsed jasmine rice, water, and salt in a rice cooker or pot
2. Cook according to the machine's instructions or until water is absorbed and rice is tender
3. In a separate pot, steam carrots and zucchini until soft, about 7-10 min
4. Fluff the rice with a fork, then gently mix in steamed vegetables and drizzle with olive oil

Tips:

- Serve this dish with a sprinkle of fresh parsley for added color and nutrients
- Ensure vegetables are steamed to a very soft consistency to be gentle on the digestion

Nutritional Values: Calories: 210, Fat: 4g, Carbs: 40g, Protein: 4g, Sugar: 3g, Sodium: 300 mg, Potassium: 200 mg, Cholesterol: 0 mg

11.2 Soothing and Hydrating

Cucumber Melon Hydration Smoothie

Preparation Time: 10 min.
Cooking Time: none
Mode of Cooking: Blending
Servings: 2
Ingredients:

- 1 cup honeydew melon, cubed
- ½ cucumber, peeled and sliced
- 1 cup coconut water
- 2 Tbsp fresh mint leaves
- 1 Tbsp lime juice

- 1 tsp honey (optional)

Directions:

1. Combine honeydew melon, cucumber, coconut water, mint leaves, and lime juice in a blender
2. Blend until smooth
3. If desired, sweeten with honey

Tips:

- Serve immediately for maximum freshness
- Can be stored in the refrigerator for up to 24 hours
- To enhance flavor, add a pinch of pink Himalayan salt before blending

Nutritional Values: Calories: 95, Fat: 0.5g, Carbs: 23g, Protein: 2g, Sugar: 20g, Sodium: 42mg, Potassium: 500mg, Cholesterol: 0mg

Soothing Herbal Bone Broth

Preparation Time: 1 hr.
Cooking Time: 3 hrs.
Mode of Cooking: Simmering
Servings: 4
Ingredients:

- 2 lb. chicken bones
- 1 gallon water
- 1 onion, quartered
- 4 cloves garlic
- 1 Tbsp apple cider vinegar
- 1 tsp turmeric powder
- 1 tsp dried parsley
- Salt and pepper to taste

Directions:

1. Place bones in a large pot and cover with water
2. Add onion, garlic, apple cider vinegar, turmeric, parsley, and seasoning
3. Bring to a boil, then reduce to a simmer and cook uncovered for 3 hrs, skimming foam as necessary

Tips:

- Strain broth through a fine-mesh sieve and discard solids
- Store in refrigerator overnight to let fat solidify for easy removal
- Can be consumed warm or used as a base for other recipes

Nutritional Values: Calories: 40, Fat: 0g, Carbs: 3g, Protein: 6g, Sugar: 1g, Sodium: 58mg, Potassium: 370mg, Cholesterol: 0mg

Apple Ginger Hydrating Drink

Preparation Time: 5 min.
Cooking Time: none
Mode of Cooking: Mixing
Servings: 1
Ingredients:

- 1 cup apple juice, preferably organic
- 1 Tbsp fresh ginger, grated
- 2 tsp lemon juice
- ½ cup sparkling water
- Ice cubes
- Mint leaves for garnish

Directions:

1. Mix apple juice, grated ginger, and lemon family health juice in a glass
2. Top with sparkling water and stir gently
3. Add ice cubes and garnish with mint leaves

Tips:

- Serve immediately to enjoy its refreshing taste
- If preferred, sweeten with a teaspoon of honey or agave syrup
- Ginger can be adjusted based on tolerance and preference

Nutritional Values: Calories: 120, Fat: 0g, Carbs: 30g, Protein: 0g, Sugar: 28g, Sodium: 20mg, Potassium: 150mg, Cholesterol: 0mg

CHILLED AVOCADO SOUP

Preparation Time: 15 min.
Cooking Time: none
Mode of Cooking: Blending
Servings: 2
Ingredients:

- 1 ripe avocado, peeled and pitted
- 1 cucumber, peeled and diced
- 1 cup plain yogurt
- 2 Tbsp lemon juice
- 2 cups cold water
- Salt and white pepper to taste
- 1 Tbsp chives, chopped for garnish

Directions:

1. Place avocado, cucumber, yogurt, lemon juice, and cold water in a blender
2. Blend until smooth
3. Season with salt and white pepper to taste

Tips:

- Chill in the refrigerator for at least 30 minutes before serving
- Garnish with chopped chives
- Can be thinned with additional water if a lighter consistency is desired

Nutritional Values: Calories: 190, Fat: 15g, Carbs: 12g, Protein: 4g, Sugar: 6g, Sodium: 60mg, Potassium: 560mg, Cholesterol: 5mg

CUCUMBER MINT HYDRATION SMOOTHIE

Preparation Time: 5 min
Cooking Time: none
Mode of Cooking: Blending
Servings: 2
Ingredients:

- 1 large cucumber, peeled and sliced
- 1 cup fresh spinach
- 1/2 ripe avocado
- 12 fresh mint leaves
- 1 Tbsp chia seeds
- 2 cups coconut water
- juice of 1 lime
- 1 Tbsp honey

Directions:

1. Combine all ingredients in a high-speed blender
2. Blend until smooth
3. Serve chilled

Tips:

- Add ice cubes for extra chilliness
- Blend on high speed for 60 seconds for optimal smoothness

Nutritional Values: Calories: 180, Fat: 5g, Carbs: 30g, Protein: 3g, Sugar: 15g, Sodium: 250 mg, Potassium: 600 mg, Cholesterol: 0 mg

11.3 SIMPLE AND LIGHT

STEAMED GINGER TURMERIC FISH

Preparation Time: 15 mins
Cooking Time: 20 mins
Mode of Cooking: Steaming
Servings: 4
Ingredients:

- 4 fillets of white fish such as cod or tilapia
- 1 Tbsp freshly grated ginger
- 2 tsp turmeric powder
- 1 lemon, thinly sliced
- Salt to taste
- Fresh coriander leaves for garnish

Directions:

1. Place the fish fillets on a steaming tray or basket
2. Sprinkle grated ginger, turmeric, and a dash of salt over each fillet
3. Top each with a few lemon slices
4. Steam in a steamer for 20 mins or until the fish is cooked through and flaky

Tips:

- Serve garnished with fresh coriander for a refreshing touch
- Pair with steamed vegetables for a complete meal

Nutritional Values: Calories: 120, Fat: 1g, Carbs: 0g, Protein: 25g, Sugar: 0g, Sodium: 75 mg, Potassium: 480 mg, Cholesterol: 60 mg

Quinoa and Roasted Vegetable Bowl

Preparation Time: 10 mins
Cooking Time: 25 mins
Mode of Cooking: Roasting and Boiling
Servings: 4
Ingredients:

- 1 C. quinoa
- 2 C. water
- 1 zucchini, cubed
- 1 bell pepper, chopped
- 1 small red onion, sliced
- 1 Tbsp olive oil
- Salt and pepper, to taste
- Juice of 1 lemon
- Fresh parsley, chopped

Directions:

1. Rinse quinoa under cold water and drain
2. In a saucepan, bring 2 C. water to a boil, add quinoa, reduce heat to low, cover, and simmer until water is absorbed and quinoa is tender, about 15 mins
3. In a separate tray, toss zucchini, bell pepper, and onion with olive oil, salt, and pepper, and roast in an oven preheated to 425°F (218°C) for 25 mins
4. Combine cooked quinoa and roasted vegetables, drizzle with lemon juice, and garnish with fresh parsley

Tips:

- Ideal for meal prep as it stores well in the fridge for up to 3 days
- Customize by adding different vegetables or a protein like chickpeas or chicken

Nutritional Values: Calories: 220, Fat: 6g, Carbs: 36g, Protein: 8g, Sugar: 5g, Sodium: 30 mg, Potassium: 560 mg, Cholesterol: 0 mg

Soft Scrambled Eggs with Chives

Preparation Time: 5 mins
Cooking Time: 8 mins
Mode of Cooking: Scrambling
Servings: 2
Ingredients:

- 4 large eggs
- 2 Tbsp milk
- 1 Tbsp unsalted butter
- Salt and pepper, to taste
- 1 Tbsp chopped fresh chives

Directions:

1. Crack eggs into a bowl, add milk, salt, and pepper, and beat until mixture is homogeneous
2. Melt butter in a non-stick skillet over low heat
3. Pour in the egg mixture, letting it sit without stirring for 1 min, then gently stir until eggs are just set but still soft and slightly runny
4. Remove from heat and fold in chopped chives

Tips:

- Avoid high heat to keep the eggs tender and creamy
- Serve immediately for the best texture and flavor

Nutritional Values: Calories: 150, Fat: 11g, Carbs: 2g, Protein: 12g, Sugar: 2g, Sodium: 170 mg, Potassium: 130 mg, Cholesterol: 372 mg

Herbal Infusion Cleanse Tea

Preparation Time: 5 mins
Cooking Time: 5 mins
Mode of Cooking: Infusion
Servings: 2
Ingredients:

- 2 Tbsp fresh mint leaves
- 1 tsp sliced ginger
- 1 Tbsp honey
- 1 lemon, juiced
- 2 C. boiling water

Directions:

1. Place mint leaves and sliced ginger in a teapot
2. Pour boiling water over the herbs, cover, and let steep for 5 mins
3. Strain into two cups, stir in honey and lemon juice to taste

Tips:

- This beverage can be consumed warm or chilled for refreshment
- Honey adds a soothing sweetness which can be adjusted to taste

Nutritional Values: Calories: 60, Fat: 0g, Carbs: 16g, Protein: 0g, Sugar: 14g, Sodium: 5 mg, Potassium: 50 mg, Cholesterol: 0 mg

Steamed Ginger-Turmeric Fish

Preparation Time: 15 min
Cooking Time: 20 min
Mode of Cooking: Steaming
Servings: 4
Ingredients:

- 4 medium fish fillets, such as cod or tilapia
- 1 Tbsp freshly grated ginger
- 1 tsp turmeric powder
- 2 Tbsp olive oil
- 1 Tbsp lemon juice
- Salt to taste
- Fresh cilantro for garnish
- Lemon slices for serving

Directions:

1. Season fish fillets with salt, ginger, and turmeric
2. Drizzle with olive oil and lemon juice
3. Place in a steamer over boiling water
4. Cover and steam for 20 min until fish flakes easily with a fork
5. Serve garnished with fresh cilantro and lemon slices

Tips:

- Serve with a side of steamed vegetables for a complete meal
- Turmeric has anti-inflammatory properties, which can aid in digestive recovery
- Ginger adds a soothing element to help settle the stomach

Nutritional Values: Calories: 200, Fat: 10g, Carbs: 1g, Protein: 25g, Sugar: 0g, Sodium: 70 mg, Potassium: 500 mg, Cholesterol: 55 mg

CHAPTER 12: 45-DAY MEAL PLAN

Embarking on a journey to manage and alleviate diverticulitis is much like learning a new language; it demands patience, practice, and a guided structure to become fluent in the signs and responses of your body. Welcome to the 45-Day Meal Plan—a carefully crafted sequence designed not just to calm and heal your digestive tract, but to reshape your relationship with food in a way that sustains and nourishes beyond mere symptom management.

This plan isn't merely a diet; think of it as a re-education of your digestive system, a gentle guiding hand leading you from the initial healing phases to a more vibrant, food-inclusive lifestyle. The next 45 days will unravel in three distinct phases. Each is constructed with the precision of a skilled artisan to ensure that you gain confidence in identifying foods that soothe, heal, and rejuvenate your body.

We begin with **Phase 1: Initial Healing**. Here, the focus is on soothing the gut, calming inflammation, and nurturing your body back from any immediate discomfort of diverticulitis. By introducing broths, gentle fibers, and hydrating beverages, we set a foundation that prioritizes healing.

Transitioning into **Phase 2**, we'll expand your culinary vocabulary. This is the period where your gut starts to adapt and accept a broader array of ingredients. The recipes become a bit more diverse, offering a delicate balance between maintaining gut health and enhancing meal satisfaction with flavors and textures that are both healing and heartwarming.

Finally, **Phase 3: Long-Term Maintenance** will mark the beginning of your onward journey with a strengthened understanding of how different foods can be safely reintroduced into your diet. This phase is designed to bolster your confidence, allowing you to maintain gut health with a more varied and enjoyable diet.

As we progress through these phases together, remember that each recipe has been developed to ensure that managing your diverticulitis is not only effective but also enriching—an approach that promises lasting health and pleasure in eating without fear. Here's to discovering how resilient and adaptive your gut can truly be!

12.1 PHASE 1: INITIAL HEALING

WEEK 1	breakfast	snack	lunch	snack	dinner
Monday	Ginger Pear Barley Porridge	Rice Cakes with Almond Butter and Banana	Chicken Bone Broth	Cucumber Rolls with Herbed Cream Cheese	Baked Lemon Herb Chicken
Tuesday	Creamy Millet and Pumpkin Cereal	Yogurt and Fruit Parfait	Carrot Ginger Soup	Ginger-Turmeric Steamed Carrots	Steamed Garlic Ginger Fish
Wednesday	Spiced Quinoa Apple Hot Cereal	Classic Hummus and Veggie Sticks	Lentil Soup	Roasted Zucchini with Parmesan and Herbs	Cumin-Spiced Turkey Patties
Thursday	Soothing Rice Porridge with Dates and Almonds	Cucumber Rolls with Herbed Cream Cheese	Quinoa and Avocado Garden Salad	Yogurt and Fruit Parfait	Lemongrass Infused Grilled Shrimp
Friday	Ginger Turmeric Oat Groats	Yogurt and Spiced Pear Parfait	Beet and Feta Sunshine Salad	Rice Cakes with Almond Butter and Banana	Herb-Crusted Baked Chicken Breast
Saturday	Banana Almond Flax Smoothie	Steamed Carrot Ribbons with Lemon and Dill	Spinach and Blueberry Vitality Salad	Yogurt and Spiced Pear Parfait	Golden Turmeric Chicken and Rice Casserole
Sunday	Spinach Ginger Detox Smoothie	Mashed Sweet Potatoes with Cilantro and Lime	Turkey and Spinach Wrap	Classic Hummus and Veggie Sticks	Hearty Vegetable Lasagna

WEEK 2	breakfast	snack	lunch	snack	dinner
Monday	Berry-Gut Healing Smoothie	Yogurt and Spiced Pear Parfait	Salmon and Cucumber Rolls	Steamed Carrot Ribbons with Lemon and Dill	Lentil and Quinoa Bake
Tuesday	Tropical Turmeric Protein Smoothie	Classic Hummus and Veggie Sticks	Veggie and Hummus Wrap	Mashed Sweet Potatoes with Cilantro and Lime	Soothing Chicken and Wild Rice Casserole
Wednesday	Banana Almond Bliss Smoothie	Rice Cakes with Almond Butter and Banana	Chicken Caesar Lettuce Rolls	Roasted Zucchini with Parmesan and Herbs	Hearty Vegetable Lasagna
Thursday	Zucchini Ribbon & Feta Egg Muffins	Yogurt and Fruit Parfait	Turkey and Spinach Wrap	Ginger-Turmeric Steamed Carrots	Savory Slow-Cooker Pot Roast
Friday	Silky Turmeric Scramble	Cucumber Rolls with Herbed Cream Cheese	Quinoa and Avocado Salad with Citrus Vinaigrette	Yogurt and Fruit Parfait	Root Vegetable Slow Cooker Stew
Saturday	Garden Veggie Steam Omelette	Steamed Carrot Ribbons with Lemon and Dill	Earthy Beet and Feta Salad with Walnut Dressing	Rice Cakes with Almond Butter and Banana	Chickpea Tagine with Apricots and Almonds
Sunday	Herbed Egg Clouds	Mashed Sweet Potatoes with Cilantro and Lime	Chicken Bone Broth	Classic Hummus and Veggie Sticks	Slow-Cooked Mediterranean Chicken

Imagine the initial phase of the 45-day meal plan as setting the stage for a grand performance, where every player—the foods you choose—has a role in calming and healing your digestive tract. As you embark on this journey, it is crucial to start with the fundamental principle of simplicity. The gut, already potentially inflamed and sensitive from diverticulitis, will benefit greatly from a diet that minimizes complexity and maximizes nurturing and healing.

In the first two weeks of Phase 1, the goal is to soothe your gut with easily digestible, non-irritating foods. Your daily meals should focus on gentle fibers and proteins, hydrating fluids, and nutrients that support healing without causing further stress to your digestive system.

Gentle Fibers

Opt for soluble fibers which dissolve easily in water and form a gel-like substance in the gut, helping to soften stools and reduce irritation. Foods such as oatmeal, ripe bananas, applesauce, and cooked carrots are excellent options. These foods help manage the pace at which nutrients are absorbed, preventing the overstimulation of the gut.

Hydration

Ample hydration is your best ally during this period. Water is essential, but incorporating herbal teas like ginger or peppermint can add soothing benefits, aiding in digestion and calming upset stomachs. Avoid caffeinated beverages as they can dehydrate and stimulate the intestines too much.

Proteins

Protein is crucial for repair and healing, but choosing the right types is key. Lean meats such as turkey, chicken, and fish cooked without heavy oils or spices, or vegetarian options like tofu and tempeh, are ideal. These proteins provide the necessary nutrients without taxing the digestive system.

Foods to Avoid

During this sensitive period, there are certain foods that can trigger more harm than good. It's advisable to steer clear of whole nuts, seeds, and popcorn as these can aggravate the walls of the gut. Also, avoid highly processed foods, which often contain additives and preservatives that can lead to inflammation. Dairy products can be problematic for some individuals due to lactose intolerance, which can exacerbate symptoms of diverticulitis, so it's wise to limit or avoid these as well during the initial phase.

Cooking Methods

How you prepare your meals is just as important as what you are eating. During this initial phase, focus on steaming, baking, or boiling rather than frying or sautéing. These cooking methods help retain the nutritional integrity of the food without adding unnecessary fats or irritants.

Listen to Your Body

Remember, the key to success in this phase is to listen to your body. Symptoms of diverticulitis can vary widely from person to person, so if a recommended food exacerbates symptoms, take note and adjust accordingly. This personalized approach helps create a diet plan that not only aims to heal but also respects the unique responses of your body.

The insights gained in these first two weeks are invaluable as they lay the groundwork for the subsequent phases of your meal plan. By following these guidelines, you're setting the best possible conditions for healing, allowing your gut to rest and recover, preparing you for a gradual reintroduction of a broader variety of foods. Each day is a step toward reclaiming your health and vitality, guided by the understanding that the right foods can indeed be your best medicine.

12.2 Phase 2: Transition to Regular Eating

WEEK 3	breakfast	snack	lunch	snack	dinner
Monday	Herbed Mushroom Omelet	Low-FODMAP Trail Mix	Quinoa & Chard Stuffed Peppers	Coconut Macaroons Delight	Seared Chicken with Ginger-Spinach
Tuesday	Savory Baked Eggs in Avocado	Yogurt and Berry Tart with Almond Crust	Barley and Mushroom Pilaf	Low-FODMAP Trail Mix	Grilled Fish with Lemon-Herb Quinoa
Wednesday	Quinoa Porridge with Cinnamon Apples	Chewy Banana Nut Quinoa Bars	Black Bean Tacos	Refreshing Fruit Sorbet	Low-FODMAP Meatloaf
Thursday	High-Fiber Blueberry Pancakes	Spiced Applesauce Cake	Lentil and Spinach Stew	Coconut Lemon Zest Macaroons	Blended Zucchini Basil Soup
Friday	Tropical Fiber Muffins	Pumpkin Seed and Cranberry Energy Bites	Black Bean and Quinoa Tacos	Ginger Turmeric Almond Flour Cookies	Ginger Poached Chicken
Saturday	Chia & Berry Sunrise Smoothie	Classic Hummus and Veggie Sticks	Fiber-Boosted Chia Pudding	Yogurt and Fruit Parfait	Carrot Ginger Puree
Sunday	Apple & Cinnamon Bran Porridge	Ginger Turmeric Almond Flour Cookies	Quinoa Apple Crisp	Rice Cakes with Almond Butter and Banana	Soft Jasmine Rice with Steamed Carrots and Zucchini

WEEK 4	breakfast	snack	lunch	snack	dinner
Monday	Herbed Egg Clouds	Rice Cakes with Almond Butter and Banana	Turkey and Spinach Wrap	Steamed Carrot Ribbons with Lemon and Dill	Lemongrass Infused Grilled Shrimp
Tuesday	Berry Smoothie Bowl	Yogurt and Fruit Parfait	Chicken Bone Broth	Mashed Sweet Potatoes with Cilantro and Lime	Herb-Crusted Baked Chicken Breast
Wednesday	Ginger Pear Barley Porridge	Classic Hummus and Veggie Sticks	Carrot Ginger Soup	Roasted Zucchini with Parmesan and Herbs	Golden Turmeric Chicken and Rice Casserole
Thursday	Creamy Millet and Pumpkin Cereal	Cucumber Rolls with Herbed Cream Cheese	Lentil Soup	Ginger-Turmeric Steamed Carrots	Hearty Vegetable Lasagna
Friday	Spiced Quinoa Apple Hot Cereal	Yogurt and Spiced Pear Parfait	Quinoa and Avocado Garden Salad	Yogurt and Fruit Parfait	Savory Slow-Cooker Pot Roast
Saturday	Soothing Rice Porridge with Dates and Almonds	Steamed Carrot Ribbons with Lemon and Dill	Beet and Feta Sunshine Salad	Rice Cakes with Almond Butter and Banana	Root Vegetable Slow Cooker Stew
Sunday	Ginger Turmeric Oat Groats	Mashed Sweet Potatoes with Cilantro and Lime	Spinach and Blueberry Vitality Salad	Classic Hummus and Veggie Sticks	Chickpea Tagine with Apricots and Almonds

As the curtains gently draw back after the initial two weeks of focused healing, the transition to regular eating in weeks three and four offers an exciting new act in your dietary journey. This phase is about broadening your dietary horizons while maintaining the care and consideration your gut has begun to appreciate and respond to positively.

During this period, the reintroduction of more diverse foods is approached with the careful optimism of an artist selecting colors for a new canvas. It becomes essential to paint your meals with a broader palette, carefully observing how each new addition affects the overall picture of your digestive health.

Broadening Fibers

The inclusion of a wider variety of fibers becomes a priority. Gradually introduce insoluble fibers which don't dissolve in water and can help add bulk to your stool. Foods like whole grains, including barley, brown rice, and whole wheat, alongside more fibrous vegetables such as kale, broccoli, and Brussels sprouts should be introduced slowly and in small quantities. These are measured steps, aimed at testing their impact while continuing to nurture your gut.

Experimenting with Fats and Proteins

This phase allows for cautious experimentation with slightly richer forms of proteins and the introduction of healthy fats. Avocado, nuts (chewed well or in butter form), and seeds can be reintroduced, observing their tolerability. Similarly, you may add small portions of red meat or eggs, expanding beyond the lean white meats and vegetarian proteins embraced in the initial phase.

Progressive Food Trials

The reintroduction should follow a structured format — introduce one new food at a time in a small amount and monitor your body's response for a couple of days. This focused approach helps in identifying any food that triggers symptoms, making it easier to adjust your diet moving forward without overarching setbacks.

Cultured and Fermented Foods

Adding cultured and fermented foods can aid in restoring and maintaining healthy gut flora. Options like yogurt (if dairy is tolerated), kefir, sauerkraut, and kimchi introduce beneficial bacteria to your digestive system, aiding in digestion and immune support. Start with small servings to see how your gut responds before making them a regular part of your diet.

Mindful Eating Practices

As you venture into more varied eating, continuing the practices of mindful eating becomes invaluable. Chew thoroughly, eat slowly, and listen attentively to the cues your body sends. This attentive relationship with eating not only enhances digestion but also increases the enjoyment and satisfaction derived from your meals.

Continual Adaptation

Emphasize flexibility in your diet during this transition phase. If certain reintroductions do not go as planned, it is important not to view this as a setback, but rather as valuable information to refine your dietary strategy. Adjustments might be necessary, and allowing yourself the room to tweak your diet ensures that the transition evolves as a sustainable practice.

Transitioning to regular eating is an enriching process that fosters a deeper understanding of your body's needs and how different foods can meet them. It's a learning curve where each meal can teach you more about your path to lasting gut health and vitality. As these weeks unfold, you are encouraged to embrace both the joys and challenges they bring, knowing each step is integral in crafting a diet that supports not only your physical well-being but also your enjoyment of life's culinary pleasures.

12.3 Phase 3: Long-Term Maintenance

WEEK 5	breakfast	snack	lunch	snack	dinner
Monday	Chia & Berry Sunrise Smoothie	Low-FODMAP Trail Mix	Quinoa & Chard Stuffed Peppers	Coconut Macaroons Delight	Seared Chicken with Ginger-Spinach
Tuesday	High-Fiber Blueberry Pancakes	Yogurt and Berry Tart with Almond Crust	Barley and Mushroom Pilaf	Low-FODMAP Trail Mix	Grilled Fish with Lemon-Herb Quinoa
Wednesday	Tropical Fiber Muffins	Chewy Banana Nut Quinoa Bars	Black Bean Tacos	Refreshing Fruit Sorbet	Low-FODMAP Meatloaf
Thursday	Apple & Cinnamon Bran Porridge	Spiced Applesauce Cake	Lentil and Spinach Stew	Coconut Lemon Zest Macaroons	Blended Zucchini Basil Soup
Friday	Quinoa and Oat Blueberry Pancakes	Pumpkin Seed and Cranberry Energy Bites	Black Bean and Quinoa Tacos	Ginger Turmeric Almond Flour Cookies	Ginger Poached Chicken
Saturday	Quinoa Porridge with Cinnamon and Pear	Classic Hummus and Veggie Sticks	Fiber-Boosted Chia Pudding	Yogurt and Fruit Parfait	Carrot Ginger Puree
Sunday	Berry Smoothie Bowl	Ginger Turmeric Almond Flour Cookies	Quinoa Apple Crisp	Rice Cakes with Almond Butter and Banana	Soft Jasmine Rice with Steamed Carrots and Zucchini

WEEK 6	breakfast	snack	lunch	snack	dinner
Monday	Quinoa Porridge with Cinnamon Apples	Herbed Mushroom Omelet	Turkey and Spinach Wrap	Classic Hummus and Veggie Sticks	Lemongrass Infused Grilled Shrimp
Tuesday	Savory Baked Eggs in Avocado	Banana Almond Flax Smoothie	Chicken Bone Broth	Rice Cakes with Almond Butter and Banana	Herb-Crusted Baked Chicken Breast
Wednesday	Herbed Mushroom Omelet	Spinach Ginger Detox Smoothie	Carrot Ginger Soup	Yogurt and Spiced Pear Parfait	Golden Turmeric Chicken and Rice Casserole
Thursday	Ginger Pear Barley Porridge	Berry-Gut Healing Smoothie	Lentil Soup	Steamed Carrot Ribbons with Lemon and Dill	Hearty Vegetable Lasagna
Friday	Creamy Millet and Pumpkin Cereal	Tropical Turmeric Protein Smoothie	Quinoa and Avocado Garden Salad	Mashed Sweet Potatoes with Cilantro and Lime	Savory Slow-Cooker Pot Roast
Saturday	Spiced Quinoa Apple Hot Cereal	Banana Almond Bliss Smoothie	Beet and Feta Sunshine Salad	Roasted Zucchini with Parmesan and Herbs	Root Vegetable Slow Cooker Stew
Sunday	Soothing Rice Porridge with Dates and Almonds	Zucchini Ribbon & Feta Egg Muffins	Spinach and Blueberry Vitality Salad	Ginger-Turmeric Steamed Carrots	Chickpea Tagine with Apricots and Almonds

In the grand tapestry of managing a condition like diverticulitis, reaching Phase 3—the Long-Term Maintenance—is akin to finding a rhythm in a new dance. It's about moving confidently with the knowledge and insights you've gathered about how your body responds to various foods and diet patterns. In weeks five, six, and seven, the goal shifts from reintroduction to establishing and refining a sustainable way of eating that balances enjoyment with your dietary needs.

Embracing Variety

Diversity in your diet is crucial in this phase. A varied diet ensures a broad intake of different nutrients, which supports overall health and helps mitigate the risk of future flare-ups. Introduce a wider range of vegetables, fruits, whole grains, and protein sources, while staying mindful of their preparation and your body's responses. This not only enhances the nutritional content of your meals but also keeps your diet interesting and enjoyable.

Strategic Eating Patterns

Focus now on how often and how much you eat. Adopting a pattern that spaces meals and snacks consistently throughout the day can help manage digestion and prevent the GI tract from becoming overwhelmed. Listen to your hunger cues and avoid overeating by serving controlled portions and eating slowly, allowing your body ample time to signal fullness.

Long-Term Fiber Integration

Having tested how your body handles various types of fiber, you are now in a good position to integrate them more fully into your diet. Aim for a balance between soluble and insoluble fibers to maintain healthy digestion and bowel movements. Sources like legumes, berries, nuts, and whole grains can be regular staples, adjusting quantities as needed based on your tolerance.

Managing Fat and Protein Intake

Fat is an essential part of a healthy diet but choosing the right types of fat is key. Incorporate sources of unsaturated fats such as olive oil, avocados, and fatty fish, which support inflammation reduction. Continue with a variety of lean proteins, incorporating plant-based options regularly to offer different nutrients and flavors while keeping the digestive system engaged but not overwhelmed.

Mindful Modifications

At this stage, with a broadened diet, occasional indulgences can be accommodated. The key is moderation and mindfulness. Should you choose to indulge in something that's generally off your list, gauge its portion size and frequency. Understanding that an occasional treat is part of a balanced life can maintain motivation and satisfaction.

Sustainable Practices

Maintaining long-term health requires not just adherence to dietary guidelines but also incorporating other lifestyle factors that support digestive health. Regular physical activity, staying hydrated, managing stress, and adequate sleep all play crucial roles in digestive health and overall well-being.

Continual Learning and Adjustment

The journey doesn't end here. Treat each week as an opportunity to learn more about your body and to refine your eating habits further. Keep a food diary to track how certain foods affect you, making it easier to identify patterns and make adjustments. Stay informed about new research into gastrointestinal health and consider regular consultations with a nutritionist to stay on track.

Phase 3 is not simply about maintenance but about thriving with a balanced, enjoyable, and health-conscious approach to eating. It's about leveraging everything you've learned during your journey to craft a lifestyle that feels as good as it tastes—a lifestyle that supports not only your gut health but also your life's pleasures and demands.

Chapter 13: Conclusion and Final Thoughts

As we approach the conclusion of this transformative journey, it feels appropriate to pause and reflect on the strides we've taken together. Understanding and managing diverticulitis through dietary changes is far from a superficial topic—it's a profound transformation that touches every aspect of your life. Throughout these pages, we've explored not just the "what" and the "how" of eating for gut health, but the "why" behind each choice, each nutrient, and each meal plan.

Managing a condition like diverticulitis is often perceived as a restrictive and solitary path, yet, I hope you've discovered it is anything but. This journey is rich with opportunities for renewal and healing, not just for you, but for your loved ones who gather at your table. From soothing soups that mend and nourish, to vibrant, fiber-rich meals that restore, every recipe has been designed to bring joy as well as healing into your kitchen.

Perhaps one of the most significant revelations may come from recognizing how interconnected our health is with the food we consume. With every fiber-rich bread and every low-FODMAP meal, you've been laying down the foundation for a healthier, more vibrant life. It's about more than soothing the symptoms; it's about crafting a lifestyle that embraces wholesome, nutritious foods as sources of both pleasure and health.

As you continue forward, remember that the journey doesn't end here. The next phase is one of sustained health and continued vigilance—a lifelong commitment to nurturing your body. Embrace this challenge with the same enthusiasm and conviction that brought you this far. With the knowledge and skills you've gathered, you are now equipped to face the future with confidence.

Carry forward the lessons learned and let them guide you to lasting health and wellness. Remember, every meal is a choice, and every food you eat can either be a step towards wellness or away from it. Choose wisely, live well, and let your food be your lifelong medicine. Keep experimenting, keep learning, and most importantly, continue this journey with the same courage and curiosity that led you to start.

13.1 Reflections on Dietary Management

In this journey of discovery and healing that we've embarked on together, the cornerstone has been understanding and managing dietary choices to best support your body through the trials of diverticulitis. As we reflect on the intricacies of dietary management, it's clear that the simple act of choosing what to put on your plate becomes an integral part of your health narrative.

The meticulous attention to diet that diverticulitis demands is not just about avoiding certain discomforts; it is, fundamentally, a proactive approach to fostering well-being from the inside out. Managing this condition compels us to look beyond the immediate pleasure of eating, to consider the longer-term implications of dietary choices on our gut and overall health.

Crafting a Thoughtful Approach to Eating

The journey starts with embracing dietary fiber — a crucial ally in your quest to manage diverticulitis. Early on, you learned that both soluble and insoluble fiber play critical roles. Soluble fiber helps to regulate digestion and can ease inflammation, whereas insoluble fiber adds bulk to stool, aiding in its transit through your digestive system.

However, the education doesn't stop at just knowing about fiber. An important lesson from our discussions has been the nuanced understanding of food tolerance, which varies widely among individuals. The introduction of the low-FODMAP diet highlighted how certain foods, while seemingly innocuous, can exacerbate symptoms for some. This personalized insight encourages a method of self-study — tracking and responding to your body's unique reactions to different foods.

The Role of Anti-inflammatory Foods

Amidst these adaptations, the anti-inflammatory foods emerge as heroes. Foods rich in omega-3 fatty acids, turmeric, ginger, and leafy greens aren't just staples of a health-centric kitchen; they embody the preventive approach that is essential in managing a chronic condition like diverticulitis. This provides you not just a means to soothe symptoms, but a pathway to long-term health optimization.

It's also important to underscore how crucial it is to stay hydrated. Water is a powerful tool in your dietary arsenal, helping to soften stool and support digestive health, which is vital for those managing diverticulitis.

Flexibility and Balance Over Rigidity

One of the more liberating insights from this journey may be the understanding that effective dietary management does not equate to draconic restrictions. Instead, it advocates for a balanced, flexible approach to eating that can accommodate the inevitable ebb and flow of life. Learning to adjust your diet in response to your diverticulitis' activity level is a skill that demands patience and insight, but one that rewards with stability and a sense of control.

The Role of Planning

Indeed, the importance of planning cannot be overstated. The 45-day meal plan is more than a schedule of meals; it serves as a blueprint for establishing a routine that can accommodate the unpredictability of your condition. This plan teaches the importance of preparation, which ensures that dietary management remains feasible and effective, even on the busiest of days.

Building a Supportive Dietary Environment

Another critical element in managing diverticulitis through diet involves creating an environment that supports your dietary needs. This involves not just the selection of the right foods, but also preparing your household—and even your social circle—to accommodate and support your dietary strategy. Communicating with family and friends about your dietary needs can help avoid the conflicts and temptations that might derail your dietary management.

Reflecting on Progress and Continuing Education

As you reflect on your progress, remember that education is an ongoing process. The landscape of nutritional science is continually evolving, and keeping abreast of the latest research not only helps optimize your diet but also empowers you to make informed decisions about your health.

The Importance of Consistency

Finally, the most crucial of the lessons learned may be the importance of consistency. The benefits of dietary management, as we've explored, are cumulative. The transformation in your health is wrought not by radical, one-time changes, but by the small, consistent choices you make every day. This consistency is what sustains your digestive health and mitigates the frequency and severity of diverticulitis flare-ups.

As you continue to navigate the complexities of managing diverticulitis, approach each day as both a challenge and an opportunity—an opportunity to heal, to learn, and to live more fully. Your diet, rich in nutrients and tailored to your personal needs, is not just a prescription, but a gateway to a more vibrant life.

In harnessing the power of food, you harness the power to reshape your health. As we close this chapter, carry forward this knowledge, not as a set of rigid rules to be followed, but as a dynamic toolkit that will evolve and adapt with you on your journey to wellness.

13.2 Sustaining Long-Term Health

Throughout our journey together in this book, we have thoroughly explored how to manage and mitigate the symptoms of diverticulitis through informed and thoughtful dietary choices. Now, as we look towards the horizon of this path, it's imperative to consider not just managing symptoms for a season, but sustaining robust health for a lifetime.

The notion of long-term health, particularly in the context of a chronic condition, can seem daunting. It often invites questions about sustainability: How can one maintain this level of dietary vigilance indefinitely? How do you incorporate these lessons into your life, so they become not just a regimen, but a part of your ethos? The answers lie not in the rigid adherence to strict guidelines, but in developing a mindset that prioritizes adaptability and awareness.

Embracing Adaptability

Life is inherently variable, fraught with unexpected changes and challenges. Therefore, sustaining long-term health involves cultivating a dietary strategy that is flexible enough to accommodate these changes. This means having the foundational knowledge to make informed choices and the creativity to adapt recipes and meals as your circumstances necessitate.

For instance, during times of remission, you might experiment with broader food choices, carefully observing how your body reacts to the reintroduction of certain foods. On the other hand, during a flare-up, returning to the basics of your 45-day meal plan provides a trusted framework that eases symptoms and supports healing.

Cultivating Mindfulness and Connection

Long-term health is deeply intertwined with a mindfulness of both the body's signals and the psychological needs that influence eating habits. This dual awareness helps in recognizing not just the physical impacts of food, but also the emotional contexts that shape eating patterns. Such mindfulness encourages eating practices that are consistently aligned with healing and health, rather than momentary indulgences.

Building a supportive community—whether it's family, friends, or fellow sufferers—also plays a crucial role in sustaining health. Sharing insights, challenges, and successes with others provides not just emotional comfort, but also practical support and accountability. This community becomes a reservoir of collective wisdom and encouragement, bolstering your individual efforts.

Regular Monitoring and Adjustment

Just as a gardener tends to their plants, checking for signs of distress or disease, so too must you regularly assess your digestive health. Regular consultations with healthcare providers, keeping a food and symptom diary, and staying informed about the latest research in digestive health are all practices that help maintain the course toward long-term wellness.

Implementing regular health assessments can alert you to changes that might necessitate a dietary shift. This proactive approach minimizes risks and empowers you with the insight to adapt your diet to continuously support your health.

Education and Advocacy

Empowerment through education is a pillar of sustaining long-term health. The more you understand about diverticulitis and its interactions with various foods and lifestyle choices, the more equipped you are to make decisions that align with health and well-being.

Becoming an advocate for your health, and possibly for others suffering from diverticulitis, transforms personal challenges into opportunities for advocacy and change. Sharing your story, promoting awareness, and advocating for better nutritional understanding can not only enrich your life but can also inspire and motivate others.

Celebrating Milestones

Maintaining motivation can often be one of the biggest challenges in any long-term health plan. It's vital to celebrate milestones along your journey—not just the big victories but also the small, everyday successes. Each day that you choose a healthy meal, each flare-up you navigate intelligently, and each new recipe you master are steps towards a healthier future. Acknowledge these achievements, and allow them to fuel your journey forward.

Continuing the Journey with Optimism

Approach your long-term dietary management with optimism. While the path of chronic disease management often includes setbacks, maintaining a positive outlook fosters resilience and adaptability. Anticipate challenges but remain focused on the potential for good days and better health.

In essence, sustaining long-term health with diverticulitis is an ongoing process of adaptation, learning, and commitment to self-care. It invites you to not only make choices that soothe and heal but to live in a way that is deeply attuned to your body's needs. As you move forward, carry with you the knowledge that each choice you make builds upon a foundation of well-being that can support not just years, but a lifetime of better health.

13.3 Additional Resources

Navigating through the complexities of diverticulitis and its dietary management can sometimes feel like a labyrinthine journey, often requiring an assortment of resources beyond individual experience and knowledge. To support your ongoing commitment to health, it is useful to extend your personal network of resources—comprising books, websites, professional associations, and support groups. These additional resources can offer not just information but also the camaraderie and support needed to manage your condition effectively.

Books and Publications

Expanding your home library with in-depth resources on gastrointestinal health is a proactive way to deepen your understanding. Consider investing in books that not only discuss diverticulitis but also broaden your insight into overall digestive health and nutrition sciences.

- **"Gut: The Inside Story of Our Body's Most Underrated Organ" by Giulia Enders** provides a captivating exploration of the digestive system, offering insights that are valuable for anyone looking to improve their gastrointestinal health.
- **"The Complete Low-FODMAP Diet" by Sue Shepherd and Peter Gibson** is an essential guide for anyone navigating the complexities of the low-FODMAP diet and provides practical advice for implementing this diet in a way that manages symptoms effectively.
- **"Fiber Fueled" by Will Bulsiewicz** offers a fresh perspective on the power of a plant-based diet rich in fiber, which can be particularly beneficial for those managing conditions like diverticulitis.

Websites and Online Platforms

The internet is awash with information, but finding credible, reliable sources is crucial. Websites run by medical institutions, certified health professionals, and patient advocacy groups can be invaluable in providing up-to-date, research-backed information.

- **Mayo Clinic (mayoclinic.org)** offers comprehensive articles on a wide range of health topics, including diverticulitis. Its content is vetted by health professionals and easy to understand.
- **The International Foundation for Gastrointestinal Disorders (iffgd.org)** is a website that provides a wealth of information on GI disorders, including downloadable resources and tools for managing digestive health.

- **Monash University's FODMAP website** and their associated app offer tools and insights that are especially useful for those following a low-FODMAP diet. Monash University is a leader in FODMAP research, and their resources are invaluable for in-depth understanding and daily management.

Support Groups and Communities

Connecting with others who are facing similar health challenges can provide not only emotional support but also practical advice that comes from lived experience. Support groups—whether online or in-person—offer a platform to share stories, tips, and encouragement.

- Local and online support groups can be found through social media platforms such as Facebook or forums dedicated to digestive health. **The Diverticulitis Subreddit** on Reddit and **Inspire's Digestive Health Community** offer active, supportive spaces for discussion and advice.
- **The Gut People (thegutpeople.net)** is a network where patients and healthcare providers come together to share knowledge and experiences related to gastrointestinal problems, including diverticulitis.

Professional Associations and Health Foundations

Associations and foundations often provide a bridge between scientific research and the lay public, offering educational resources, community programs, and the latest research findings that can help you stay informed about the best practices in health management.

- **The American Gastroenterological Association (gastro.org)** offers not only professional resources but also patient-directed materials that can help in understanding the options and treatments available for gut health.
- **The Crohn's & Colitis Foundation** may focus primarily on IBD, but it also offers extensive resources on broader digestive health issues, including community events and patient education programs that might be of interest to those with diverticulitis.

In utilizing these resources, remember to approach them as tools in a larger kit designed to give you control over your health. They should serve not only as sources of information but also as sources of comfort and community. As you build and broaden your understanding of diverticulitis and dietary management, let these resources empower you with a sense of advocacy for your health journey. Engage actively with the content, ask questions, and seek clarity—this proactive engagement will serve you well in your continued pursuit of health and wellness. Whether through books that deepen your understanding, websites that offer the latest research, or support groups that provide a sense of community, these resources are invaluable companions on your path to sustained health.

www.ingramcontent.com/pod-product-compliance
Lightning Source LLC
Chambersburg PA
CBHW081553250726
48653CB00009B/3406